POLITICAL
MALPRACTICE

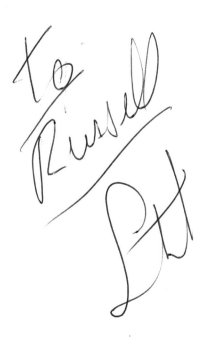

How the Politicians
Made a Mess of Health Reform

POLITICAL
MALPRACTICE

Stanley F. Hupfeld

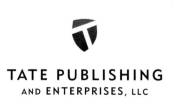

TATE PUBLISHING
AND ENTERPRISES, LLC

Published by Tate Publishing & Enterprises, LLC
127 E. Trade Center Terrace | Mustang, Oklahoma 73064 USA
1.888.361.9473 | www.tatepublishing.com

Tate Publishing is committed to excellence in the publishing industry. The company reflects the philosophy established by the founders, based on Psalm 68:11,
"The Lord gave the word and great was the company of those who published it."

Book design copyright © 2012 by Tate Publishing, LLC. All rights reserved.
Cover design by Shawn Collins
Interior design by Nathan Harmony

Published in the United States of America

ISBN: 978-1-61862-292-1
1. Health & Fitness / Health Care Issues
2. Political Science / Commentary & Opinion
12.01.18

Dedication

I was indeed fortunate to have married "the girl next door." My wife of more than forty years, Suzie, is an extraordinary person. She is my perfect example of the virtue of tolerance. If I can follow her example, I find I am a better human being.

After all is said and done, and we, as Shakespeare says, "shuffle off this mortal coil," we are ultimately to be judged by our children.

Our three children, Matthew, Kelly, and Kate, are wonderful parents, spouses, and citizens. Our grandchildren, Travis, Turner, Evie, Cami, Annie, and Claire are fortunate to have these extraordinary people as parents. If for no other reason, the legacy of our children and grandchildren means Suzie and I have been extraordinarily successful.

Since my typing skills are practically zero, I have enlisted the aid of my very capable assistant, Suzan Nesom Whaley, who has patiently typed every word of this manuscript as I sat by her desk and dictated to her from a handwritten version. This is, without a doubt, old school writing.

Acknowledgments

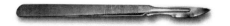

My sincere thanks go to the many very smart people who have advised and consulted with me on the ideas presented in this book. Thank you to Lyn Hester, Beth Pauchnik, Bill Wandel, Lynn Horton, Dr. Nazi Zuhdi, Dr. Jim Long, Dr. Charles Bethea, Dr. Mary Ann Bauman, Susan Relland, Dr. Rocky Fredrickson, Dr. Mary Stefl, Jeff Greene, Marshall Snipes, Zora Brown, Kim Holland, and John Delano.

Special thanks go to a group who read the final version of this manuscript and added some very special recommendations to make it more readable and logical. They include: Hadley Ford, Mike Fogarty, Rich Umbdenstock, and Greg Meyers.

Also, thanks to M. J. Van Deventer, a former journalism professor who provided great help editing this manuscript.

It's been my privilege to work for the last twenty-three years for an extraordinary Board of Directors at INTEGRIS Health. Their vision, sense of history, and passion for doing the right thing are exemplary.

Finally, my special gratitude goes to the doctors, nurses, technicians, and staff members with whom I've work over the years. They toil, often unrecognized, every day to make the health and the lives of the patients they serve just a little better.

Table of Contents

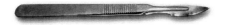

Foreword

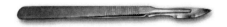

When Stan Hupfeld asked me to write the forward to his book, I was honored. Stunned, but honored. As the CEO of the largest network of proton radiation therapy centers in the world I am very well known by the approximately five people who have heard of proton therapy. Stan, however, is a recognized leader in healthcare, not just in Oklahoma where he recently retired as CEO and President of INTEGRIS Health, the largest hospital system in the state, but regionally and nationally. He has served on the Board of Directors of the American Hospital Association, and is the former Chairman of the AHA's Regional Policy Board, as well as Chairman of the INTEGRIS Family of Foundations. He was also a running back for the Texas Longhorns when they won a national championship, and is a Vietnam veteran. Wherever he goes, excellence follows. He has more letters after his name than I have in my name. I am proud to call him my friend and mentor.

I first met Stan six years ago to talk about how, together, we might change the delivery of cancer care in Oklahoma. INTEGRIS Health had a good cancer program, but Stan, in typical Stan fashion, wanted to make it the best. My company offers a unique form of cancer treatment that Stan recognized would dramatically change the care patients in his state would receive. He didn't hesitate in pursuing his vision for a new, state-of-the-art, comprehensive cancer center with proton therapy as the anchor. He wanted to make sure patients in Oklahoma, and the broader region, had access to the same level care they would have at M.D. Anderson or Mass General. We have worked closely together ever since. His vision was recently recognized when Health Leaders-InterStudy, a leading provider of managed care market intelligence, reported that Oklahoma City is quickly becoming the medical tourism destination for oncology care in the United States. He is one of the most visionary healthcare executives I have worked with, and definitely one of the most humble.

I have always enjoyed Stan's observations on healthcare. I have found him to be frank, pulling no punches, and over laying his comments with a dry and wicked sense of humor. He also writes a monthly column that I read religiously. So, when he told me he was writing a book, I was excited to see what he would have to say (and to see if he would grow a ponytail). I haven't been disappointed. He uses his almost 40 years of healthcare experience as a lens through which to bring into focus the problems which exist in healthcare today. Right up front Stan poses the question of "what is the very best health system we could devise that would routinely deliver a high quality of care at reasonable costs to the most people?" This seems like a goal that anyone who is drawn to healthcare would be proud to pursue. But Stan admits that in his career he was influenced by the unintended consequences of the incentives in our healthcare system in ways that took him away from that simple goal. This is a remarkable admission for a healthcare executive. It foreshadows a book filled with keen insight on human behavior, and provocative and nuanced observations of the actions we all take based on how we are rewarded.

He has written a book for anyone wanting a straightforward explanation of why healthcare is the way it is in the United States. He strips away the rhetoric of the political sound bites and looks at the incentives that have been woven into our healthcare system, and the consequences that have resulted, both intended and unintended. It is a book that makes you stop for a moment and think. And that is something more people need to do if we are ever to fix our current system. However, I still think he would sell more books if he grew that ponytail.

—Hadley Ford
CEO
ProCure Treatment Centers

Preface

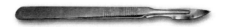

Have you ever wanted to throw something at your television set? I have. During the 2010 debates over health reform, I came very close to executing my flat screen. Watching politician after politician drone on incessantly about how "Obamacare" was either a godsend to the American public or the worst social legislation to ever befall it, my exasperation level rose to new heights.

It is clear to me neither side had a clue how to deal with the major domestic issue of our time. The night the *Patient Protection and Affordable Care Act* passed, out of frustration I arose at 2:00 a.m. and wrote a column that eventually our daily newspaper, *The Oklahoman*, published. In this article, I excoriated the leadership of both parties for ill-serving the American public.

My frustration has only risen since that night as the repeal debate has taken shape. Once again, my television set is at great risk of termination. I found the only thing that could satisfy this demon within me was to write about how and why politicians on the nightly news just had it wrong.

This small book is a result of that exorcism. Since I am so critical of both parties, it is a fair question to ask about my own particular political philosophy. My attempt at an even-handed criticism of both sides should provide some clue. However, further explanation may be helpful.

To explain myself, I must go back to my own history.

My father landed on Normandy Beach a week after D-Day. I understand even after seven days it was still a fairly scary undertaking. I was born in July 1944 while he was slogging it out in the fields of France. He ultimately won a Bronze Star for bravery.

Unfortunately, I was not smart enough to ask him about his experiences before he died. The only references I recall him making to the war were his expressions of respect for Dwight D. Eisenhower when he ran for president in 1952. He clearly loved this man.

Eisenhower led my father, and millions of others, in the largest amphibious invasion in the history of the world. As a consequence, he was a huge supporter of "Ike" and thus, the Republican Party. He also thought Eisenhower's opponent, Adlai Stevenson, was a wimp.

Clearly, as a result of this experience, Eisenhower became one of my favorite historical characters. So much so I would reference him years later any time I was asked to speak on leadership.

After my father passed, I found in his effects pictures he had taken at the front in France and Germany. One of these pictures was of Joe Louis, then heavyweight champion of the world, who at that time was visiting the troops.

My favorite was a picture of Winston Churchill, also visiting the front and reviewing the troops as my father snapped his picture. I've had a lifelong fascination with Churchill. This fascination is based on Churchill's unabiding belief in his own ability. Even though he was in his sixties when he rose to the world stage as a prime minister of England at the beginning of World War II, he never lost faith in his destiny. Finding that picture was indeed a treasure.

My father was a smoker. He was addicted to cigarettes through the U.S. Army. The military apparently provided these death sticks to our soldiers and sailors, unwittingly addicting a whole generation. My father died in his early sixties as a result of lung cancer and associated heart disease.

My mother was a nurse. In fact, she met my father in a Baltimore hospital while taking care of his mother. My mother was perhaps the toughest and most resilient person I have ever known. During my early years, she was a school nurse in the Dallas School System. While working full time and taking care of her family, she would make an eighty-mile round trip drive to Denton, Texas, three times a week for years while getting her bachelor's and master's degrees in counseling.

She ultimately became a school counselor and finished her career as a grade school principal. Her greatest frustration in forty years with the Dallas School System was attempting to fire an incompetent teacher. She had to fight the teacher's union every step of the way. It took two years and left her exhausted and bitter.

My mother loved John Kennedy and loathed Richard Nixon. She died twenty years after my father. She was in her eighties at the time. My experiences with her long deterioration into dementia have shaped many of my frustrations with the medical care system. My concern of how we deal with our elderly is clearly influenced by that exposure.

As an only child growing up in Dallas in the 1960s, I was aware of all the cruelties of segregation. I went to Catholic schools and played football at Jesuit High School. Since I was in a Catholic school, I had several black teammates.

In the 1960s in Texas, white kids could not play against black kids in the public school system. Since half of our games were against public schools, my black teammates could not play. In fact, since we played in public stadiums, they could not even get into the gates. The only time they were allowed inside the stadium was when they had a football uniform on and we were playing another private school.

As a result of some success as a small, slow running back, I received a football scholarship to the University of Texas. I was fortunate enough to be a part of the 1963 National Championship team. Even though I was not a good enough player to ever see action, I have a championship ring and lots of memories. As I live longer and memories fade, I am gradually becoming a very good player.

One of my strongest memories is that of the Kennedy assassination in November 1963. Like all of us at that time, I remember exactly where I was standing when I heard the news Kennedy had been shot.

I also remember practicing that day. We were undefeated at the time and had one more regular season game against Texas A&M to complete a perfect season. Despite this tragedy, it was, after all, Texas, and football is king.

I graduated with a degree in History and English. I remember my father was convinced I would probably never get a job with that kind of fuzzy degree.

After a brief try at dental school—I was not very good with my hands—I became a Medical Corps Service Officer in the army and ultimately went to Vietnam. It was there I learned, even though I would never touch a wounded soldier, that if I did my job reasonably well I could make the caregivers'—in this case the medics'—job easier.

With that inspiration, I went to graduate school in health care administration. In graduate school, my thesis focused on a prediction that we would have national health insurance in the next few years. This was 1970.

So much for my predictive abilities.

After graduate school, I began my love affair with managing the health delivery system and the intricacies of health policy. For almost forty years, I was the chief executive officer of either an American hospital or health system. Just as in Vietnam, I found if I did my job well, I could impact the care delivery process, and I could help make the jobs of those whose privilege it was to care for patients more productive.

For the past fifteen years, I have written a monthly column on health policy for a local daily business journal in Oklahoma City, *The Journal Record*. I have received encouragement from many of my friends and colleagues to take my writing to the next level. It seems this book is an outgrowth of that encouragement. It was also an opportunity to remove real mortal danger to my television.

So my politics? Since the common wisdom is that you vote your pocketbook, I, by all rights, should be a Democrat. After all, the Democrats have always been predisposed to help human service providers, such as hospitals, more than Republicans.

However, it seems to me the Democrats have sold their souls to trial lawyers. I have been a part of lawsuits through the years where abuses by the plaintiffs' bar are extraordinary. As you will see in the following pages, my view is our tort system must be changed, but probably not for the reasons you might expect.

In Oklahoma, you must register to vote by party. I am a registered Republican and, therefore, cannot vote in Democratic primaries. But, in the general election I do not hesitate to vote for a superior candidate if they are Democratic.

In politics, I would describe myself slightly right of center. By the way, this is exactly where I believe most of the American public resides. I am very frustrated by the Democrats' capitulation to trial lawyers, union bosses, and extreme environmentalists. Equally, I believe the Republicans have it wrong on many social issues. Although, as a Catholic, I believe abortion is wrong, I do not accept it being a litmus test for electability.

For the last several years, I've chaired an organization known as the Fit Kids Coalition. We have successfully passed legislation to change what children eat and drink in public schools. At each step of the way, we have fought and overcome the blockheads who insisted no one could tell our schools what to do.

That very freedom, of course, is what got us into this mess in the first place. Oklahoma ranks near dead last among the states in the obesity level of its citizens.

I point out in future sections that hospitals have little or no incentive to engage in public health activities. Nevertheless, I am proud my organization has taken a leadership role in many public health initiatives. Our leadership has recognized health has more to do with where people live, what they have to eat, and particularly how well educated they are than anything our doctors and hospitals can do.

In order to fulfill its mission to make a difference in our community's health, we have accepted this global view of health and have been able to put together some extraordinary programs. One of which I am most proud is a charter school we operate. As the only health care system in the United States to actually operate a public school, this effort required extraordinary vision by our board. We've taken the full legal and financial responsibility for the operation of a kindergarten-through-fifth-grade elementary school, with a population of approximately 90 percent African Americans and almost 100 percent poverty. Virtually every child is on the school lunch program.

During the past ten years we've operated as a charter school, the academic performance of these children has increased significantly. We've demonstrated that these children, coming from sometimes the most difficult of backgrounds, can learn as well as their more affluent neighbors *if* provided the right nurturing environment.

As I retired from my position as Chief Executive Officer of INTEGRIS Health, I was honored to have the school named after me. My grandson, Travis, correctly noted, while he was happy for me, he was confused because how can you have a school named after you if you're not dead?

Two virtues I attempt to emulate are those of balance and tolerance. Growing up in a household of very different political points of view, I always have been influenced by the need to see both sides of any argument. I have little regard for politicians or public figures who think they are smarter than the rest of us and whose ideology is so fixed that any thoughtful discussion of alternative points of view is impossible. I hope I can take the best ideas from divergent views and encourage common-sense solutions.

The second virtue I strive to emulate is that of tolerance. My early days on the football fields of Texas, trying to come to grips with the injustices of segregation, has clearly influenced my desire to see the best in people, appreciate their differences, and encourage their development.

As you read my thoughts on health reform, it should become abundantly clear that my sense is neither side of the political aisle has served us well. Perhaps we can expect nothing more from a group whose primary purpose is to position themselves for their next election.

I will attempt to explain why changing our system of health services in the United States will be so difficult to achieve while at the same time outlining what must be done to create a health system that better serves us all. As you will see, my main thesis is we already spend sufficient money on our health care system to cover millions of currently uninsured without raising taxes or creating a new entitlement. To do so, however, will require we have the moral and political courage to make changes that will make some elements of our current system very uncomfortable. In fact, the disagreements this book may engender encourage me that I am on the right track.

Right or Privilege

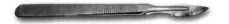

God never read the Declaration of Independence.

~ William Durrant

While many of us believe in a God who loves all of us equally, clearly we are not all created equal. We are endowed individually with far different DNA. This difference makes some of us brighter or more athletic or even better looking.

Some of us will simply live longer and enjoy a healthier life. This genetic protection that some of us enjoy and others do not means some of us will have far greater need for the services of our health system than others. This need begs the question, "What right do we have to access that system?"

Ever since Harry Truman proposed universal health coverage as he prepared to run for the presidency in 1948, the question of health care as a right or a privilege always seems to surface. I hardly ever attend or speak at a gathering interested in this issue without that very question being raised. Having tried on numerous occasions to answer it intelligently and having been a total failure, I have concluded it is indeed a trick question.

If you answer it is clearly a right, then you must be prepared to define that right and from where that right comes.

- Is it God-given?
- A natural right we have as a human being?
- Or does our Constitution grant this right to us?

As either a God-given, natural, or constitutional right, it must be defined. Since those who suggest it is a right clearly are not implying that we all have the right to good health, as God allows us all to eventually get sick and die, they must mean we have a right to health care services.

Every right needs to be defined lest it be rendered unrecognizable. Thus, our right to free speech is limited by the prohibitions against slander or yelling fire in a crowded theatre. So, too, our right to health care must be defined.

- Do we all have the right to plastic surgery or to Viagra if someone else pays the bill?
- Do we all have the right to a lung transplant if our own behavior—smoking—irreparably damages our lungs?
- Does the emergency or the nature of the need affect or impact our right to acquiring that service?

Said another way, is our right to health care services limited to basic primary and emergency care, or does it extend all the way to esoteric or even cosmetic treatments? The point is, the claim that health care is a right must be accompanied by a definition of how much health care is included in that assertion.

Equally perplexing is the argument that health care is a privilege.

Privileges are grants by one entity or person to another entity or person. Doctors have privileges at hospitals. Their medical degree or state license does not automatically entitle them to practice medicine in that facility. They have no inherent right to that opportunity except that granted by the hospital after review of their training, experience, and intellectual and moral integrity to deserve that privilege.

The privilege also can be removed for failure to live up to any hospital's standards.

If access to health care services is a privilege, who is the grantor of that privilege? Is money or social standing the sole determinant of this privilege? Privilege granting implies a grantor of the privilege and criteria for that award. In both circumstances, failure to award that privilege to the least among us would offend our inherent spirit of egalitarianism or even our Judeo-Christian ethic.

So the answer to the conundrum of *is healthcare a right or a privilege* is that it is both.

It is a *right* because, legally, we have treated it as a right. Every hospital is obliged to see every patient who walks in its door.

It is a *privilege* because no doctor is obliged to see patients they care not to have in their practice.

It is a *right* because we believe in our bones the poor deserve compassion and health care in times of need.

It is also a *privilege* because we believe in our bones no one has the right to call on the unlimited resources of a health care system irrespective of their personal need or economic circumstance.

The health care debate in the past several years has been fueled by high-sounding rhetoric and low-brawl obfuscations. It has not, however, been marked by intellectual and thoughtful discussion around highly profound and, in some cases, deeply troubling complexities.

This book is an attempt to have an adult conversation about these complexities in a way that examines the nuances of the issues that were largely lost in the partisan political rumblings we tend to hear on the network and cable news of all stripes.

My effort here is not to take sides on what has become a frenzied debate over whose sound bite wins the day but is an examination of the underlying issues that get lost in partisan bickering. My effort here is to have a conversation that touches the elements of health policy often ignored because of the noise level of political rhetoric.

So, for instance, this book discusses how we treat our elderly and how we differ in this from the rest of the world without getting stranded by accusations that are somehow a subterfuge to deny the elderly their needed end-of-life care.

Then, we will move to a discussion about our recently passed new health reform law from the perspective of how some would like to change what has been a uniquely American health care system to one more similar to a Western European–style system.

If we accept that our plan must be as appropriate to future needs as our current system is unique to our values and culture, then this book concludes with some distinctly American solutions.

Finally, perhaps it is important to tell you what this book is not. It is not a detailed blueprint for health reform. It is about changing incentives to get a different result.

At the advent of World War II, Congress gave President Franklin D. Roosevelt the ability to freeze wages as the country went into an austere wartime economy. As a result of these restrictions, unions turned to negotiating over benefits, especially a relatively new benefit called health insurance.

Created only a decade earlier, health insurance was a relatively cheap throwaway for companies to provide. Thus stimulated with very low deductibles and insatiable patient demand, the medical industry exploded. Now, seventy years later, we have the highest-cost health system in the world.

We have physicians and hospitals incentivized to provide high-cost technological solutions to virtually every medical problem.

We have a pharmaceutical industry that advertises directly to consumers over the heads of the physicians who do the actual prescribing of their product.

We have an insurance industry that is motivated more by their stock portfolio than the need to pay medical claims.

All these incentives will be explored as we describe how they not only stimulate our trillion-dollar system but actually impact the choices we and our doctors make.

These changes are not easy. In fact, several are quite difficult. They are intended to take complications out of the health system. My premise is that some change is necessary. The suggestions I make are intended to reset the dynamics of a complex system in a way to facilitate a common-sense approach.

I began this book with the assumption that the goal of covering more people while improving quality and holding costs relatively constant is still the primary objective of the entire reform discussion.

Implicit in this assumption is that overly simplified solutions, such as the problem can be solved by selling health insurance across state lines, or as overly complicated as the several-thousand-page *Patient Protection and Affordable Care Act*, are wrong for the same reason. Neither side addresses the incentives already deeply imbedded in our system. These incentives drive a mindset and a culture, which, unless recognized and addressed, will ultimately doom any reform plan.

As we shall see, there are already sufficient dollars in the system to accomplish the goal. Significant new taxes are not needed. Armies of bureaucrats are not needed. Even overly simplified jargon about market-based solutions is not needed.

All that is needed is the will to change, the will to redirect decades of incentives that drive some excellent health care but also come with limited access and high cost.

Throughout these discussions, we must never forget the role of the caregiver, most especially the physician, and how he or she can adapt to the new world order.

One final note before we begin our journey into the convoluted world of health delivery and the incentives that drive it. Nothing I will point out is intended to criticize anyone's behavior, with the possible exception of our politicians. Individuals, hospitals, doctors, and insurance companies are simply responding to the built-in incentives our system promotes. My belief is that if we are to get a different behavior, we simply must change these incentives.

What Makes American Health Care Unique?

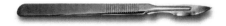

> For every complex problem there is an answer
> that is clear, simple, and wrong.
>
> —H. L. Mencken

On Valentine's Day 2009 Tina Chumbley was wheeled
into an operating room at INTEGRIS Baptist Medical
Center in Oklahoma City to receive a donated kidney. That same day her daughter, Jennifer, was taken to
another operating room at INTEGRIS Baptist to donate
a kidney. What made this special was that Jennifer was
not giving her organ to her mother but to a stranger, Scott
Clark, who was being prepared in a third operating room.
Scott's sister, Cindy, was in yet another operating room
at INTEGRIS Baptist having her kidney harvested for
shipment to Barnes-Jewish Hospital in St. Louis while
Scott waited for a kidney to be sent from Johns Hopkins
in Baltimore. This was all part of a 12-patient, three-state
and three-hospital domino kidney transplant, the nation's
first six-way domino kidney transplant effort.

The press release that day stated, "Kidney paired dona-
tion (KPD) takes a group of incompatible donor-recipi-
ent pairs and matches them with other pairs in need of a
compatible kidney. By exchanging kidneys between the
pairs, it is possible to give each recipient a compatible kidney. Each recipient receives a kidney from a stranger and
transplants are enabled that otherwise would not have
taken place. Involving multiple hospitals created even
more possibilities for matches.

"In the domino swap, a surgical team made up of nine
surgeons, six anesthesiologists and 12 nurses began a cross-
country set of operations with five incompatible pairs. An
altruistic donor and a recipient who was next on the United
Network for Organ Sharing (UNOS) organ recipient list
started and ended the domino. Altruistic donors are those
willing to donate a kidney to any needy recipient.

"Just like falling dominoes, the altruistic donor kidney
went to a recipient from one of the incompatible pairs,
that recipient's donor kidney went to a recipient from a
second pair, and so on. The last remaining kidney from
the final incompatible pair went to the UNOS recipient.

"As part of this complex procedure, Johns Hopkins
flew one kidney to INTEGRIS Baptist; INTEGRIS
Baptist flew one kidney to Barnes-Jewish, and Barnes-
Jewish flew one kidney to Johns Hopkins."

This is a first-rate example of the sophistication of
American medicine. Miracles such as these happen com-
monly in American hospitals, performed by brilliant
American physicians, aided by skilled nurses using world
class technology.

At the same time, only a few miles away from Baptist, some of the world's most desperate people lined up quietly to receive free health care from volunteer doctors and nurses working in a free clinic. Though most of these individuals were employed, they had no health insurance for them or their families. They hoped the clinic's meager resources would address their pressing health needs. If they were lucky, nothing urgent would be discovered that could not be resolved by small doses of medication dispensed by the clinic's undersized pharmacy. If they were not so fortunate and more comprehensive care was needed, they must wait while the clinic attempted to persuade volunteer specialists and a hospital to take on their case at no cost. This process could take weeks or even months. This is the high and the low of medicine in this country. This is where we must start our journey of understanding.

The obvious salient question is what would be the very best health system Americans could devise that would routinely deliver high-quality care at reasonable costs to the most people?

As a hospital chief executive officer for almost forty years, I thought I was answering that question every day. In retrospect, I was probably driven by the incentives inherent in our health system to maximize my hospital's reputation, market share, and bottom line. While these are not unreasonable actions, especially for someone paid to produce results for my employers, I submit they probably have little to do with answering the main question.

It is a surprisingly simple question, so simple it is stunning we can get no agreement on the answer. If our market-driven approach, which is the basis of the American system, is unsatisfactory and if we are equally unsure whether a Western European–type solution works for us, then what is the alternative, and why does it seem to elude us?

If I am right that access to health care services is neither a right nor a privilege but ultimately some of both and not totally much of either, this could explain why the American system has been so resistant to change.

The rest of the world became comfortable with the governmental-based approach decades ago. The American system now stands alone as unique among the world's democracies in its approach to health care. This uniqueness will not give way easily, and even now, with the passage of reform legislation, change will be slow, difficult, and painful. Thus, our system deserves a dispassionate look at the forces within the system that will resist any substantial change.

First, while the concept of private insurance is known in much of the world—even those with highly regimented nationalized systems—the coverage of the majority of the working population by private insurance is a singular American invention.

From the early days of the first Blue Cross plan in the 1930s, our health insurance industry has experienced tremendous growth. The idea of your employer paying for the majority of your health costs through a subsidy of its workers' health premiums is deeply ingrained in our psyche. It drives many Americans to choose their employment based on the richness of their employers' health coverage.

This passing of the risk for the cost of care from the employee to the employer has had a significant effect on the delivery and use of health services. In short, the multiplier effect on costs is breathtaking. A simplistic but nevertheless accurate analogy may be in order.

I give my daughter, Kelly, my credit card and instruct her to go to the mall and buy anything she thinks she wants. Once there, she hands my credit card to the sales person and requests they select for her anything they think she needs. What would be the impact on my next credit card statement? It is obvious. My cost would be out of control. I am paying the bill. My daughter is receiving the benefits of this buying spree, and the sales person enhances their sales commission.

This is a complete disconnect between the ultimate responsible party, the recipient of the goods or services, and the person selecting the product. The acceleration on the cost borne by the cardholder is exponential.

This, in essence, is our private health insurance system and essentially the reason cost increases are explosive. The economic disconnect between the patient, the doctor, and the payer condemns us to a high-cost solution to every problem.

Second, we are using a basically incorrect term to describe our system. The term *health insurance* on its face is a misnomer. In classical terms, *insurance* is the taking of a small amount of money from the many to cover the losses of the few.

When we purchase homeowners' coverage, it never occurs to us to expect our insurance carrier to reimburse us when someone throws a ball through our window. In Oklahoma, we are plagued every spring with tornadoes. If one were to destroy my home, I would certainly expect my policy to protect me.

However, our expectation in regard to our health insurance is that every contact with a health system gets paid in whole or in part by our carrier. By classic definition, this is not insurance. It is a transfer-of-payments device. The insurance company takes money from the employer and passes it to the provider and takes a percentage cut as the money moves past them.

Their underwriting risk is substantially less than that borne by, for instance, a property and casualty company. Since we began with incorrect terminology and a system skewed to high costs, it is little wonder we wind up with a system that defies any effort to change it.

If that is not enough, there are other numerous "uniquely American" elements that make our system very difficult to change. These include:

Our Tort System

On December 7, 2010 a five-year-old girl was wheeled into an operating room of a major teaching center. She was there because a CT scan of her head had revealed a large area of bleeding with massive swelling of the brain. The neurosurgeon operating on her found significant bleeding from a very large "arteriovenous malformation" (AVM). Unfortunately, the little girl died shortly after the surgery. It was determined post mortem that the AVM was probably an inherited abnormality.

Two days earlier the young girl had been taken by her parents to a hospital emergency department (ED) due to the sudden onset of headaches, nausea, and vomiting. The emergency department doctor diagnosed gastroenteritis and assumed she would recover with a few days rest in the hospital. He did not order a CT scan as it was his judgment, later confirmed by other ED experts, that it is extremely difficult to differentiate lethargy from the effects of vomiting and fatigue in a young child in the middle of the night from something far more profound. Later that evening a floor nurse continued to chart the child as being "lethargic and unresponsive." The nurse did not report her findings to the attending physician, in this case the ED physician, because they appeared consistent with the diagnosis of gastroenteritis and lethargy. The ED doctor expected that a child of this age would naturally feel "puny" after a bout of consistent nausea and vomiting. In addition, her white blood cell count was elevated, which was consistent with a probable viral infection.

By the morning of the next day the young girl's symptoms were significantly worse and a CT scan did reveal the brain swelling. This prompted the subsequent surgery.

The family sued and claimed the ED doctor was negligent in not recognizing the early symptoms of internal bleeding which an immediate CT scan would have uncovered. This would have led to earlier surgery and possible recovery. Even though it was clear this anatomic anomaly was almost impossible to diagnose given the presenting symptoms, the hospital settled, recognizing that the sympathy engendered by the loss of a child could possibly cause a significant jury award in favor of the parents. What is important to note here is that the medicine and science were clearly on the side of the hospital, yet they were unwilling to take a chance on a sympathetic jury with distraught parents who just lost a child.

This tragedy is an isolated case taken from actual files that serves as an example of the difficult position our tort system often places on providers of health care. Emotions often matter more than facts, and physicians are often put in untenable positions. In this case the ED physician is accused of not ordering an expensive diagnostic test even though there was nothing in the physical examination that would have warranted such a procedure. It is the fear of just this sort of second guessing that drives much of the cost of care we see today.

The theory of recovering and compensating for losses due to medical mistakes or incompetence is not totally unknown to the rest of the world. It is safe to say, however, that its use and abuse in the United States has reached astronomical proportions. Essentially every doctor treats every patient as a potential litigant.

The multiplier effect on cost is incalculable. The cost of malpractice coverage for the provider is striking—and largely unknown to the rest of the world. It is, however, the hidden cost of excessive treatment that really distorts the U.S. health economy. A September 2010 Harvard study, "Medical Liability Systems," puts the cost of defensive medicine at $45 billion per year.

What is interesting is that medical malpractice lawsuits—for failing to order a test or procedure resulting in a misdiagnosis—are a relatively small fraction of the number of overall lawsuits. Generally, hospitals and doctors get sued when they make a mistake. Getting sued for missing a diagnosis happens far less frequently. The problem is, as long as physicians think they could get sued for being too conservative, they act on that belief, and that stimulates the overuse of expensive tests and procedures.

Ask any physician or health executive what is the one thing that must be changed in our system to bring cost under control; they would respond without hesitation: tort reform.

They would, of course, be correct. The Harvard study documents what they intuitively know to be true. But here is the irony: health providers benefit from our out-of-control medical legal system.

As we shall note, our fee-for-service payment system rewards and incentivizes medical providers to do as much as possible for patients. The more we do, the more we get paid.

Since the fear of litigation serves as a motivator and a stimulant to excessive diagnostic tests and treatments, and since the providers of those tests and treatments ultimately benefit financially from this excessive overuse, the thing we fear the most—being sued—actually works to our benefit.

This irony leads to the speculation if we eliminated malpractice reform tomorrow, the majority of the $45 billion of defensive medicine would not go away. Without changing the financial incentives, simply reforming the tort system is only a half measure but a necessary one.

When the financial incentive for physicians inherent in our system is added to the fear of lawsuits, then this overuse of high-cost solutions to every problem becomes endemic.

The sad fact is that people get hurt in our medical system. The legitimate concerns of these injured patients must be addressed, and compensation should be awarded when the medical system fails to protect those entrusted to its care. Our system, however, is more about addressing the needs of the litigator than that of the injured party. I have suggestions on how to insure fairness for the injured while eliminating incentives for abuse.

History of Entrepreneurship

To get a complete picture of how our system differs from the rest of the world, one must understand the mind-set that has to prevail for the assumption that access to health services is a government responsibility. In this case, health care must be viewed primarily as a social service.

As a social service, citizens have an expectation these services will be provided for and financed by the government just as police and fire coverage are provided. Clearly in the United States, access to some services, or for some people, gives us the impression health care is a social service.

We expect that with our tax dollars we will be provided with fire service if our house is burning. We, however, do not expect that our tax dollars will buy us flame-retardant building materials or fire detectors. We clearly understand the limits of a tax-funded social service.

One example is the function of the hospital emergency room. Here the expectation, both morally and legally, is that everyone who enters the doors of these facilities gets some level of diagnostic or treatment services regardless of their status or ability to pay. In Medicare, our older generation expects health services to be financed by the balance of our population.

Medicare is a perfect example of why we must exercise great caution in jumping to easy solutions for health care delivery. Medicare, when founded, was built on a very simple concept—that of providing seniors with necessary end-of-life care. In those years, people at sixty-five were generally out of the work force and uninsurable. Providing coverage for them for their later years was reasonable. However, this very provision of care has allowed the elderly to live longer, thus destroying the actuarial assumptions on which the program was originally based. With seniors living twenty to thirty years beyond retirement, the unintended consequences of this entirely reasonable gesture is an entitlement program that promises to help bankrupt the country.

The peculiarities aside, the business culture and sense of entrepreneurship surrounding our health care is again uniquely American. It is possible to find private hospitals elsewhere in the world, even in the most socialized environments. Nowhere else, however, is there a thriving hospital industry with publicly traded companies competing on the stock exchanges for the favor of investors. These companies fret over last quarter's earnings and market expectations just as any other corporate conglomerates.

The second major entrepreneurial differentiator is our pattern of physician ownership. In many parts of this country, physicians routinely own the means of medical production. Doctor ownership of diagnostic technology, MRIs, CT scanners, PET scanners, and ultrasound is common.

Also common are physicians profiting from treatment and testing operations, such as radiation facilities and even hospitals. Thus, health services in this country are both a social service and a business enterprise, and, in many cases, a very profitable enterprise.

Arguments for and against this ownership are largely philosophical in nature.

The defenders would point to our free market economy, which encourages private investment. They would note the physician expertise ensures a high quality of service.

The detractors would argue there is something unseemly about the ability of a physician to direct patients to a service from which the doctor profits individually. In a study for "Medical Care Research and Review" (August 2007), Professor Jean Mitchell of Georgetown University notes, "the introduction of financial incentives linked to ownership coincided with a significant change in the practice patterns of physician owners." Professor Mitchell found after studying workers' compensation data in Oklahoma that there was over a 2,000 percent increase in the number of expensive spinal surgeries performed after the surgeons acquired ownership of a specialty hospital.

It is this inherent conflict of interest in prescribing the very services that profit the physician that seems the most troubling. Let me return to the analogy of my daughter with my credit card at the mall. Only in this case the sales person not only gets a commission on everything she sells to my daughter, but she actually owns the dresses she is proposing. Should our understanding of human nature tell us anything about the sales girl's incentive?

Add to these differentiators our medical device and pharmaceutical industries, both of which have a stake in insuring the use of high-cost technology.

One gets a sense of the hill that must be climbed to effectively change this system.

Interwoven into this aggressive business culture is a very dynamic not-for-profit system of health care. The majority of hospitals in the United States are not for profit. These include hospitals run by some division of local or state government such as university medical schools or hospitals owned or operated by county or city governments. This category also includes hospitals started by religious organizations as a way to bring converts to their particular religious affiliation. Many of these not-for-profit systems are multi-state and or multi-billion-dollar operations. Often their business culture is every bit as competitive and aggressive as their for-profit counterparts.

These systems usually have no connection to their competitors in similar geographies. Their leadership is traditionally judged by how well their hospitals perform financially. This leads to tremendous duplication of services as each tries to capture more physician loyalty and a higher percentage of the patient dollar.

In even relatively small communities, it is not uncommon to see several sophisticated programs, such as open-heart surgery, all operating at marginal capacity with marginal clinical results.

This is true because no single hospital is willing to give up—either because of ego or economics—this profitable business. There is no incentive for hospital executives to work together to address community needs such as infant mortality or immunization rates. These executives get paid to outperform their competitors.

Pride and money force hospitals and their boards to consider only what advances their bottom line and reputation, not what would improve community health.

I was fortunate to work for a board that saw the mission of our organization in the broadest of contexts. Our goal was "to improve the health of the people we serve." Running good hospitals was necessary to help meet our goal, but it was not sufficient. They viewed health in a grander vision.

Health has more to do with where people live, what they have to eat, and most important, how well educated they are. The board encouraged management to act on that grand vision. Therefore, we established free clinics, programs for gang members, and even a charter school in an economically deprived area.

But all of these were possible only because we were successful at managing the business of running hospitals and, therefore, had the resources to invest in these community endeavors.

It was clear to me that ultimately I would be judged and rewarded by how well our hospitals performed financially, and not by the breadth or scope of our community activities.

In other words, at the end of the day, my compensation was based on our financial performance. As long as our margins stayed strong, I would be allowed and encouraged to pursue this broader vision.

Backward Economics

The sometimes-acrimonious debate over physician ownership of hospitals invariably involves discussion of the place of market-based economics in health care. The free marketers hold that only with open, unfettered markets will the U.S. ever get control of cost, aligned with optimal patient choice.

Thus, the root question is, does market-based economics work in health care?

In its most simplified form, market economics works best when competition drives down cost and raises quality. As an example, four gas stations on one corner guarantee price competition and make the operators improve service as they strive to take business away from the other three competitors. In fact, experience seems to indicate that four MRIs on a street corner drive the price up.

The reason for this? We are dealing with a relatively uninformed consumer who generally places total faith in their referring physician. The ultimate question we all have for our doctor is, "If this is your mother [substitute father, sister, child], what would you do?"

If the physician recommends a particular magnetic resonance imaging (MRI) machine, in which they may have an ownership interest, of course, that is exactly what you will select.

The gap between a physician's knowledge base and that of even his most intelligent patient is very wide. The consumer is, for all intents and purposes, uninformed and dependent. So, in our example, there is no price competition because we have an unknowledgeable and an uninformed consumer. Four MRIs on a street corner guarantee price increases.

Health care simply does not respond to the normal laws of the market place.

In a market economy, the provider of a good or service has incentives that usually line up with those purchasing their product or service. The manufacturer who produces a high-quality product for a competitive price gets a reward with customer loyalty. This same manufacturer can produce a lower-quality product with a lower price point and take the risk some consumers will be willing to trade price over quality.

After all, some of us buy a Kia; some buy a Lexus. We make a conscious choice between quality and price. Some consumers will reward manufacturers for their quality. Some people will reward them based on price.

In health care, there is no such distinction. First, the physician's incentive system is exactly the opposite of the patient's best interest. Patients want the most time with their physician. The doctor's incentive is to spend as little time as possible and then move on to the next patient.

The patient's interest is in acquiring only the absolute necessary care consistent with adequately and thoroughly addressing their immediate problem. The doctor's incentive is to do the most for the patient, consistent with maximizing their income stream. Surgeons get paid to operate, not encourage watchful waiting.

Thank God, many of our physicians do not act on what is clearly in their best financial interest. The point is, our health system definitely encourages the opposite behavior.

Second, consumers would be loath to make the price-versus-quality decision. We would resist knowingly accepting an inferior quality service for a price break. Who wants a one-time offer of discounted heart surgery with just a few of the frills eliminated? For our own health care, we all want the best—particularly since we all are usually only paying a fraction of the cost.

Our tort system demands it, and our culture emphasizes it. Those who promote health reform based on a market focus would state: *If* we are spending our own money, we would reward quality and punish the lack of it. *If* we were knowledgeable consumers and *if* we alone were making the decision, this might be true. As we have seen, neither of these is accurate.

Our View of Death

We routinely engage in medical activity for our elderly that has no parallel in the rest of the world. It is not uncommon to operate on aged patients for palliative relief of symptoms when their life expectancy is the same with or without the surgery. In short, we do things to the elderly that do not even receive discussion in the rest of the world.

There is an old sarcastic saying that the rest of the world views death as inevitable. Americans view it as optional. While a bit overdone, there is some truth in this comment. It is a well-known fact that, as Americans, we spend an extraordinary amount of money on healthcare in the final months of our lives.

It has been estimated one-half of all of our lifetime health expenditures will be spent in the last six months of our lives. Often this is to keep our parents in a semi-comatose condition in an ICU while the children decide when to let Mom or Dad go. As a culture, our inability to deal with death logically exacerbates cost problems and limits our ability to have a serious discussion about end-of-life issues.

This is really hard and serious stuff. Talking about the subject of death and end-of-life care in the abstract, and in theory, is far different than when it affects our family.

At the age of seventy-five, my father-in-law was diagnosed with prostate cancer. Studies have shown that by that age approximately 70 percent of men have the likelihood of having some degree of this cancer. In fact, more men die *with* prostate cancer than *of* prostate cancer.

Despite my father-in-law's beginning dementia and the fact his life expectancy was the same with or without the surgery, the urologist convinced my wife's family to allow him to perform a total prostatectomy. He survived and lived several more years. However, he never fully recovered from the anesthesia, and his dementia was significantly magnified.

Should the surgery have been performed? Would the decision have been different had the family been required to bear some of the cost? In fact, would the family have asked a whole different set of questions if there had been economic consequences to their decision? Even posing these questions makes us uncomfortable, but ask them we must.

The most egregious demonstration of this limitation was the focus over "death panels" during the 2010 Congressional national debate on health reform. Every conversation about the wisdom of our current medical practices relative to the elderly was met with incendiary rhetoric that this was simply a smoke screen to deny the elderly needed care.

Variation

President Obama, early in the debate over health reform, said we would only pay for "what works." No one could argue with the logic of spending only our own, our employer's, or our tax dollars on tests, procedures, and treatments that actually add value to the care process.

How this is accomplished and who makes the decision on what works is, of course, the difficult part. Historically, it was easy. Your personal physician made the decision. Whatever he or she prescribed was delivered and paid for without question. Unfortunately, it could be argued that very freedom is what got us into our current health care mess.

The differences in diagnostic patterns, surgery rates, and treatment options across the United States are huge and largely unexplainable. It is hard for the layman to understand how a profession based on the highest of scientific principles can tolerate this kind of significant variation, often on populations with relatively consistent demographics.

It appears what happens to you as a patient is in part driven by the age of your physician, where they went to medical school, and even if they have a financial interest in the diagnostic or treatment technology.

It has been speculated by the *Dartmouth Atlas* that the only consistent variable that explains these regional differences is the number of specialists and amount of high-tech facilities in each region.

For instance, if a particular region has significantly higher heart catheterizations and cardiac stents per capita than another region, then the reason seems to be there are more cardiologists and catheterization laboratories per capita in that region. This is true after all other variables are held constant. Said another way, more doctors and more new technology generate more costly solutions to medical problems than would be seen in areas with fewer of each.

Health insurance companies often find themselves as the arbiter of paying for "what works." However, this has never been a role that has been particularly important to them.

In graduate school, my health economics professor often used the maxim "in health care, what gets paid for gets done." In other words, medicine is often driven by what reimbursement standards exist in any particular community.

For instance, the delivery of medical chemotherapy has moved from the medical oncologist's office to the hospital and back again depending on where the most favorable reimbursement exists. The use of open-heart surgery versus the use of stent technology varies by which physician specialty seems to benefit the most. Heart surgeons for years worried that cardiologists were being too aggressive in the use of stents to open blocked blood vessels. Heart surgery enjoyed a resurgence when cardiologists became owners of heart hospitals and the payment for bypass surgery was significantly superior to that of placing stents. Medical treatment follows the money.

Historically, insurance companies have had the luxury of being agnostic on most treatment decisions made by physicians. Because of relatively little underwriting risk, insurance companies have little incentive to identify clinical decisions that have little or no scientific evidence to support them. Health insurance carriers could simply pass the cost of this year's expensive—and perhaps unproven—therapy into next year's premium base. There was little regulation that prevented it, and the market was clearly not price sensitive.

Under health reform, the game changes. There will be limitations on how much of the premium dollar can be devoted to overhead and profit. It is clear state insurance commissioners, and even the federal government, will initially attempt to jawbone carriers from announcing significant premium growth.

In the past, carriers have not had to pursue claims adjudication with any great sense of urgency. Yes, there were occasional media stories that often led to works of fiction about greedy health insurance companies taking advantage of sick patients. Insurance companies often would delay payment to doctors and hospitals while they dithered around asking for increasing amounts of patient data. These delay tactics irritated providers who believed they were simply clever devices to enhance the time value of the insurers' investments at the expense of the caregiver's cash flow.

However, in the grand scheme, the arrangement between carriers and providers worked relatively well for all concerned. The doctors and hospitals were paid with regularity, the insurers assumed relatively little risk, and the patient, for the most part, had relatively all of their bills paid.

As a result of increasing emphasis at the state and federal regulatory levels, health insurers are reexamining their role and are only paying for what is clinically justifiable. Since the good old days of automatic premium increases may be coming to an end, insurers now have a much greater need to keep costs in control if they expect to maintain their margins.

This new pressure to more closely examine and reimburse only scientifically-supported treatment options is exacerbated by their new requirements to cover preexisting conditions and eliminate lifetime reserves.

Failure to Communicate

Our inability to have adult discussions concerning what works also leads us to some curious practice patterns in terms of screening tests. For instance, we have accepted without question that after a certain age men get a PSA to detect prostate cancer, and women get a mammography to discover breast cancer. What does not get discussed is the relatively high level of false positives for these exams.

Based on these inaccurate results, further diagnostic (biopsy) tests or treatments are begun. This additional testing or treatment involves expense and risk. Every treatment carries with it some risk of patient injury. We have these standards for yearly testing that are supported by physicians, hospitals, equipment manufacturers, and even philanthropic health organizations, including the American Cancer Society, which ultimately benefit from this standardization.

- Does mammography uncover breast cancer that might have gone undetected? Absolutely.

- Does the requirement for yearly testing lead to unnecessary further testing and treatment? It certainly appears so.

- Can we have a thoughtful conversation about when and how often to use population-based screening tests?

Sadly, it appears we cannot.

The mere suggestion we examine these standards is met with outrage from all with vested interests.

Cost Shifting

Ever since our parents taught us there is no such thing as a "free lunch," we have understood ultimately someone pays for every good or service received. George W. Bush, while president, made the observation we really already had national health coverage for everyone. It is called the hospital ER.

Opponents greeted this with howls of incredulity as another example of his limited intellectual capacity. However, in a sense, President Bush was exactly correct. Hospitals are required to accept all comers and must at least examine each patient and initiate treatment if the condition is deemed an emergency; in essence, the uninsured do have a source of care financed by someone else.

In most industrialized nations, this source of payment is the government using tax dollars. In the United States, this source is the holders of health insurance policies. Every few years, insurers negotiate with health providers about the terms of their inclusion in the insurer's network. Of course, these terms include the payment providers will receive for their services. Part of the hospital's cost base for which they expect recognition in their payment rates is the cost of this free care.

The insurers, in turn, then build that cost into their premium structure. So while the rest of the world supports care for the poor through tax dollars, we do it through our premium payments. Some part of every medical bill, whether as part of our private portion or part of the premium dollar, is financing the expense of this cost shift.

Unclear Expectations

Each American is special and unique. We honor our individual freedoms and prerogatives more than any country in the history of the world. The tone for recognizing the importance of the individual was set in the Declaration of Independence when Thomas Jefferson wrote it is "self-evident, that all men are created equal" (at the time he meant all white men who owned property), "that they are endowed … with certain unalienable Rights…"

Our founders led us to a culture that places the individual's needs supreme over group or societal needs. The supremacy of the individual has been codified by our economic system that stresses the individual's ability to prosper based on their own motivation and work ethic. It could be argued this cultural focus on the individual is what distinguishes us as Americans and makes us the envy of the world.

This focus on the individual drives all elements of our culture. Our tort system suggests all individual grievances must be addressed, even if the cost to the rest of us is significant. Witness our medical dramas played out on television. The tenor of most of these is there is no price too high to pay to save one human life.

This egalitarian worldview leads us to the assumption each of us can and should access every bit of medical armamentaria that is available, regardless of the cost, regardless of our chance of recovery, and regardless of whether our own behavior generated the problem in the first place.

In this last instance, I am referring to cutting edge, costly therapies with sometimes marginal results made available to lifetime smokers suffering with lung cancer, and expensive life saving brain surgeries performed on motorcyclists who refuse to wear protective helmets. The point here is that the focus on our individual rights handed down by our founders has contributed to our greatness, but also acts as a barrier to coming to grips with solving our health crisis.

Most of the rest of the world is very comfortable with the fact there are times (especially at the end of life) when doing less is more humane to the individual, but also more appropriate to constraining health costs for the rest of us. In Great Britain, for instance, they actually calculate how much any treatment will cost versus how much value they put on one human life for one year. Any treatment that does not meet that threshold is denied. This sounds so very foreign and bizarre to us. I suspect the reason is our culture for the last 200-plus years has emphasized that human life is priceless. Trying to reduce it to a dollar figure somehow seems unnatural.

As a nation, we have never quite figured out how we feel or what we believe about the level of public support for the medically underserved. What is the level of care every American gets by simply being an American?

Historically, it had been decided in our national policy that every American child gets a kindergarten through twelfth grade education simply by the virtue of being an American. This is our national standard, which is usually financed by some combination of state and local taxes. It is understood and accepted as a national priority.

We are comfortable. The quality of schools, the physical condition of the schools, what we are paying teachers, or even if there is a modern football stadium are all subject to the vagaries of a tax structure for each state and school district.

We elect local school boards to administer our schools as well as account for the impact of widely different levels of economic support. Yet, the commitment of K-12 education never varies.

We, of course, have no similar agreement on what level of health care every American gets by virtue of their citizenship. There has been no attempt to define where the commitment to each of us starts or ends. We are apparently comfortable with the fact parents can make the economic decision to send their children to private school if they choose and can so afford.

This does not change the national commitment of thirteen years of education for every child for free. We are comfortable the educational experience varies directly with the socio-economic circumstances of the neighborhood in which the child lives.

Nevertheless, the commitment stays the same. Do we not have to reach the same level of commitment for each of us in terms of what slice of health care service each of us gets as a result of our citizenship? As in education, do we not have to define with some precision where our access to health services begins and ends?

If the analogy holds true, our prerogative is to take advantage of this commitment to free care or to buy up as we do in education. This is a choice we all would make. Said another way, what is the comfort level in stating Americans get a defined level of health care—basic, primary, secondary, ER visits. The system will provide anything else at your own expense.

Is health care so unique, so controversial that it defies this kind of definition? For without this definition, we are only left with the politics of who has the largest megaphone, as we will see in the next section.

Politicians as Caregivers

Every year, in almost every state legislature, there is a battle over what should be mandated to be covered in health insurance policies sold in that state. The antagonists in this battle tend to be on one side; the business community that opposes mandates because of its accelerator effect on health premiums is on the other side.

Its opponents, the ones carrying the signs in demonstrations around a state capitol building, are the individuals or relatives of those who suffer with the particular malady currently not covered. Their arguments are valid and often highly charged. Their intent is to elicit an emotional response to an economic problem.

The very idea that the treatment for autism, for instance, is not a covered service is offensive and unexplainable to them. The point is not really whether autism should be a covered problem but that this particular group might get their way if they have enough political muscle. If they are successful, the cost of autism is then borne by the policyholders and not the parents alone.

In the above section, we speculated over whether we could define a national commitment to a certain level of care for all Americans. The challenge would be that wherever the line is drawn, some group would find it objectionable because it fails to include their particular issue or need.

So just as the parents of an autistic child want to expand what insurance policies must cover, lobbying groups of all ilk will challenge any artificial line that attempts to define what we can get at the public's largesse. Anything from stomach stapling to plastic surgery for cosmetic reasons will be fair game for those who clamor for a more expensive and expansive government role in health care.

High Overhead Costs

The contention of American health system detractors is that proportionally we have significantly higher administrative costs than any system in the rest of the world. Every doctor's office and every hospital has an army of people whose sole job is to collect receivables from a plethora of insurance companies and government programs.

Each of these companies has their own requirements and specifications to access their individual collection processes. These vary widely in the amount of data required for payment. Government programs such as Medicare and Medicaid—or even less frequently billed agencies such as the Indian Health Service or Champus for military personnel—adds another layer of complexity to the receivable management process.

This variety in claims management requires painstaking adherence to each company's or agency's requirements. Since the rest of the world either has a single-payer system or not-for-profit insurance carriers, the job of getting paid is simply much easier. It is estimated the added cost of this enormous collection effort adds somewhere between 15 and 20 percent overhead to our system.

When the additional overhead is added to the assumption of 30 to 40 percent for unnecessary tests and procedures, our system could approach 50 percent of cost not experienced in other democracies across the world.

Let me again return to my daughter, Kelly, at the mall. Now that she and the sales person have collaborated on her wardrobe, I get the bill. The retailer has paid a small fee to the credit card company for a quick turnaround on their money. That fee is clearly part of the cost I am to pay. Suppose, instead of only a handful of credit card companies that the retailer accepts, they had to deal with over one hundred companies, and instead of a quick turnaround on their money, it took months. Now I am paying 20 percent more than actual cost for the dresses. That is a description of the impact of insurance on our medical system.

American Expectations

Perhaps the most intriguing and difficult part of selling health reform to the American public is their high expectations around the easy access to highly sophisticated technology.

If you need a CT scan to confirm a particular diagnosis, chances are the health system can make that happen within a few hours.

Need heart surgery? How about tomorrow morning?

Our abundance of hospitals, high-tech diagnostic centers, and outpatient services of every stripe is a great gift to those who possess some sort of insurance coverage.

This gift comes with a very high price tag. The duplication of every manner of treatment and diagnostic technology adds significant cost to our delivery of health services. Since price is mostly irrelevant in health decision making, all those MRIs, CTs, PTs, all those cath labs, open heart centers, and all those radiation treatment centers tend to get used enough to keep them viable.

But because return on investment, capital acquisition costs, and depreciation are built into the price for service, our ease of access to every manner of technology enhances the cost of our system exponentially.

Since access is so easy and quick, our expectations for immediacy of service run deep. Most of the western European health systems to which we are often compared in no way match the distribution or the abundance of our technology. This lack of access leads to waiting times. Americans are not good at waiting. Many of the comparison nations started their more centralized systems decades ago. Technology was significantly less sophisticated than today, and two World Wars left their populations with a scarcity mentality that made waiting for service more acceptable.

Today, while the sophistication of technology in Western Europe and Canada might equal the United States, the spread and availability of it is significantly different. Thus, the old charge there are more CT scanners in any large American city than in the whole country of Canada has a ring of truth. Actually, this lack of access is one reason that, in any comparison between us and similar nations, our costs, whether per capita or a percentage of the GNP, are significantly higher.

Here is how it works.

In most of the rest of the world, pricing through budgetary control is highly centralized. This keeps margins for providers low or nonexistent. With small margins, the ability to accumulate capital is severely limited. Health care, by its nature, is capital intensive. With no capital generating capability, the opportunity to replace old technology or to acquire the latest technology is very limited.

This leads to a scarcity of technology of all sorts, which alternately leads to less access then leads to waiting times. And so, one of the principle control mechanisms for the rest of the world—lack of capita—would fly in the face of American expectations. Changing our population's expectations is clearly part of the problem in moving us to a more controlled health care system.

Lack of Continuity

In the debate over health reform of care delivery, several examples of successful models were bandied about by Congress and by President Obama. The Mayo Clinic was often cited as an example of how very cost-effective medicine with great results could and should be practiced. Mayo has for years been studied and admired as the nirvana of intelligent health care delivery.

What makes Mayo so different from the way medicine is practiced in the rest of the country?

First, its doctors are not private entrepreneurs. They are employees of the clinic, and their incentive system is built around clinic success both financially and clinically. Private entrepreneurs by definition, which comprise the vast majority of American physicians, have as their main focus the maximization of their own convenience and income.

Conversations with other doctors about their patients' conditions and treatment options are time consuming and not very financially rewarding. A private physician's only product is time. Any use of that time that does not produce revenue only limits the private physician's income-producing capacity.

Look at the medicine cabinet of any elderly patient. You will see medicines of all varieties, many with negative reactions to each other, prescribed by different physicians who rarely communicate with each other. Talk to patients in hospitals with complex diagnoses who are often frustrated by the conflicting advice of various specialties who never seem to arrive at the patient's bedside at the same time.

All too often, these physicians talk only to each other about their patient via an occasional cryptic note in a medical record. There is no forum and no incentive for physicians to consult and collaborate with each other about an individual patient's condition. On top of all this, our data systems between doctors' offices, hospitals, and outpatient clinics are usually from different vendors with different levels of sophistication and with little or no ability to interface.

Even the most conscientious physician is hard pressed to determine his or her patient's past test results, medical procedures, and medication without relying on the patient's memory.

Contrast this with the Mayo model—salaried doctors with incentives that are based on patient and clinic success. In this model, the incentive system rewards—in fact, demands—physicians collaborate. There is no advantage for any doctor to maximize his or her own schedule or time to the detriment of his or her colleagues. As more physicians see employment as an option, the model of physician entrepreneurship is indeed dwindling.

How does this time maximizing work? Let's take an active surgery department in a busy private hospital any-where in the country.

A surgery department thrives on how quickly it can move patients through the surgery process. Turnover time in each operating suite is vitally important to the surgeon. Since the efficient use of their time converts to income for the surgeon, he or she needs to start and complete their operations on time.

When surgeons book operations, they estimate how much time it will take to complete the procedure. If the surgeon underestimates the completion time, that surgical suite will run late the rest of the day. If the surgeon arrives late, that room will run behind.

The fact that other surgeons are inconvenienced, or the delay throws the operating room staff into an over-time situation, is interesting but not necessarily relative to the offending surgeon. As a private entrepreneur, the physician's main interest is in maximizing his or her own efficiency. The fact their behavior may sub-maximize another surgeon's efficiency or that of the operating room staff is irrelevant.

More and more, physicians are looking for employ-ment opportunities as lifestyle becomes more important than income. The opportunity to build collaborative models with different incentives that promote collegiality should get us closer to the Mayo model.

Medicine's Secret

The dirty little secret of American medicine is the huge disparity in physician incomes. A pediatrician with relatively the same number of years of training makes annually one-tenth of what a busy neurosurgeon might make—$100,000 compared to $1,000,000.

Before we examine why, let me explain my prejudice.

I believe physicians should be the highest paid of all professionals. The competition to get into medical school is intense, and only the brightest among us succeed. Four years of medical school are followed by another four to eight years of postgraduate training under the most rigorous of circumstances. While colleagues in law and engineering have completed their training and are developing their careers, physicians are still toiling away in residencies and fellowships, usually marked by a mound of debt. The other professions have years of income production before physicians ever get off the starting block in beginning their career. If we believe hard work and preparation deserve reward, then surely physicians should be the highest paid among us.

But within the medical profession, multiples of five to ten times what some physicians earn, as opposed to others, seems a bit odd. Why? The answer is, in part, historical and in some part reflects reimbursement methodologies.

When the original Blue Cross/Blue Shield plan started in the 1930s, the control of reimbursement philosophy was seized by the surgical specialists. Their natural inclination was to reward those specialists who actually did things to patients—operate, read an X-ray, insert a catheter. They found it difficult to calculate equivalent value for spending time with patients.

Primary care physicians, often referred to as generalists, including family doctors, internal medicine physicians, and pediatricians, spend most of their time visiting with patients, conducting physical examinations, recommending diagnostic tests and procedures, and generally acting as a patient's advocate.

Time is their only product.

Historically, spending time with patients never seemed to matter quite as much as operating on them. The financial disconnect between specialists and generalists has continued to promulgate itself through the years.

This income difference is a self-fulfilling prophecy. There has developed between specialists and generalists a status difference, as well as an income difference. Medical schools historically are run by those with specialty training who subtly continue this discrimination.

The brighter medical students have more choice as to what field of medicine to enter. Would the best and brightest choose pediatrics and struggle to make one hundred thousand dollars per annum when becoming a neurosurgeon would bring one million dollars a year and significantly more prestige?

So there is little wonder those residencies that promise handsome income rewards fill first, and many family practice residencies struggle to meet their quotas. Disproportionate income and status have led, through the decades, to a shortage of primary care physicians.

This shortage will become more severe with the population blip of the aging of the baby-boom generation. As this group reaches their senior years and their health naturally deteriorates, the need for primary care services will exhaust our already depleted manpower pool of generalists.

When we add all the new entrants who now have insurance cards, the disparity of primary care physicians versus specialists will become acute.

Hospitals as Part of the Problem

In 1999, the hospital world was rocked by the Institute of Medicine's report titled "To Err is Human." This report noted adverse events that caused significant harm, and even death, to patients in hospitals accounted for 2.9 to 3.7 percent of all hospital admissions.

Extrapolating that percentage to the total number of hospital admissions in the United States meant there were forty-four thousand to ninety-eight thousand deaths every year as a result of hospital errors.

This was a staggering number that served as an embarrassment to the hospital community. This trusted symbol of American medicine, through sloppiness, inattention to detail, or plain neglect, was responsible for thousands of deaths of patients entrusted to their care.

While the human cost of these adverse events was incalculable, the dollar cost also was staggering. These mistakes cost between seventeen and twenty-nine billion dollars every year to repair. This figure does not include the cost of medication and other errors that occur in venues such as pharmacies, outpatient clinics, or doctors' offices.

What was worse, the report charged hospitals had very little incentive to change. The more mistakes they made, the more they had to fix, and thus, the more they were paid.

Unfortunately, the whole medical liability issue exacerbated the problem. Hospitals simply did not want to talk about their mistakes for fear of generating a malpractice suit. As a result, there was neither private disclosure to the patients and their families nor public disclosure to their communities. Hospitals were simply comfortable with an unsuspecting public.

This report sent shock waves through the hospital industry. Hospital leaders had to suddenly face the fact there was a shocking lack of a safety culture in our facilities. Not only were hospitals negligently causing the deaths of too many Americans, they also were contributing a huge part of the cost problem conundrum that was beginning to shake the confidence of the American public.

In summary, there are at least 14 reasons that answering the question, "How do we devise a health system that guarantees high quality and contains cost?" will pose an arduous task. This combination of vested interest and American uniqueness will continue to challenge policy makers. Our view of the world, our expectations, and the history of our medical system all provide barriers to thoughtful solutions. We ignore our peculiarities as Americans at the risk of failure.

Our Words Are
Our Problem

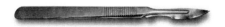

> It is the mark of an educated mind to be able to
> entertain a thought without accepting it.
>
> —Aristotle

Why was it necessary to review the litany of the uniqueness of the American system before we looked at the logic
of our current health reform legislation? Did we need
that review to determine what is suspect, what might just
work, and what we could and should suggest as an alternative to the current legislation?

The answer is really quite simple.

Any attempt to impose a system that fails to at least
consider our culture, our expectations, our tort system,
and the economies in our system is doomed to a troubled
start and maybe ultimate failure.

Frankly, I do not think failure is an option. Too much
is at stake. Too many people depend on wise decisions
being made. So we will pivot to what is admittedly a naive
assumption that we can have an intelligent discussion

about the simple question, "How do we provide quality care to the most people at reasonable costs?"

To do so, however, our rhetoric must change. We must stop saying things just because they have become convenient, seem to fit our political philosophy, or because our knowledge of the subject is so superficial the words have become comfortable alternatives for our failure to shed any meaningful light on the subject. These are partisan phrases that only serve to stifle debate.

- The first of these ill-thought-out slogans is, "We have the best health care system in the world." We indeed have great technological capability. We have some spectacularly good hospitals. We have some marvelously advanced medical schools and thousands of skilled and compassionate doctors.

  But what in the world justifies us saying we are the best? It is true many from all over the world come here to seek care. Our centers of excellence, such as Johns Hopkins in Baltimore, clearly inspire the wealthy of the world to beat a path to their door. To say the United States system is the best has to be a bit of hyperbole.

  The detractors of the United States' system in Congress and the media are equally guilty of overstatement. During the formal debate over health reform, there were consistent referrals to the United States' poor standing on major health statistics among the nations of the world. Our national life expectancy, neonatal mortality rates, and the percentage of people with untreated diabetes were examples pointed out as a symptom of a failure of our health system.

Those outraged by this poor performance would then make the case the United States is only number one in terms of per capita spending on health. Former United States Senator Tom Daschle makes this point by suggesting the U.S. spends more and gets worse results than any other major nation.

This argument ignores the fact health has as much to do with environmental factors as it has to do with the efficiency of health services. The fact is, those countries with whom the United States is compared have more extensive tax-funded social services such as education, welfare, and food, all factors that clearly impact their nation's performance relative to health performance.

Without a standard of measurement, the United States cannot justify claiming we are "the best system in the world." Similarly, lambasting our system for its relatively poor showing in several major statistical categories fails to recognize health in its most integrated form. The fact is the U.S. is excellent in certain high-tech areas. We also have many gaps in our system into which the poor and underserved often fall.

The problem with either claim is it forces the debaters into a position where an even-handed discussion becomes difficult. To claim our country is the best implies any change would only detract from that superior position. Thus, any recommendation for improvement only gets met with a chorus of, "Why should we fix what isn't broken?"

To argue we have failed on the world stage of competition suggests success would only mean duplicating the system of our more successful competitors. This then fails to take into consideration those elements that make the American system unique and difficult to change.

What should not be forgotten about many of the foreign health systems that are held up as worthy of emulation is they were started at a time when technology was much simpler and with a significantly more compliant population.

- The second phrase that limits any intelligent discussion is, "Health care decisions should only be between you and your doctor." This statement has obvious appeal. We want to believe we are in control of health decisions about our body, influenced only by the opinions of our informed and caring personal physician.

  Of course, this is pretty much how our system has worked for the past century. Where has this philosophy led us? Double-digit health inflation is in part what we have received. We must remember both parties to this equation have economic and personal motivations that have nothing to do with constraining costs.

  A physician's economic incentive is to do as much for the patient as possible, consistent with their fears of getting sued and practicing good medicine. The patient in general is not normally vested in the economic consequences of their medical decisions. Thus, if cost containment is an end goal, then we must examine the premise that health care decisions can only be between doctor and patient.

This is tricky territory. We all want a warm and trusting relationship with our doctors. I am not suggesting we lose that element of trust. I am just suggesting there must be a change in incentives for both parties or new boundaries set that bring a measure of discipline to the relationship, or both.

Let me explain.

In the 1990s, Health Maintenance Organizations (HMOs) were an attempt to reset the incentives of the physicians. Rather than a reward system that encouraged doing as much for the patient as possible, the HMO reward system was to do as little as possible consistent with keeping the patient healthy.

The HMO would take the financial risk for the total care of the patient for a defined period of time. They would get a flat fee for taking this risk. If the cost of the patient's care for that period of time was less than the fee, the HMO made money. If the cost was more, the HMO incurred a loss. This moved the financial risk of care from the payer—Medicare or the employer—to the HMO.

In this scheme, the HMO's incentive was to keep the patient healthy and avoid high-end costly solutions, such as hospital stays, if possible. What is interesting is the heyday of HMOs was the first time in decades inflation in health cost was less than inflation of the general economy. HMOs simply worked.

However, HMOs were not well liked. Many patients distrusted them. There was a perception medical decisions were being made on their behalf based on generating a profit for the HMO rather than what was in the patient's best interest.

Many patients did not like the sense of when they could see a specialist and what procedures could be done—controlled, in many cases, by a primary care doctor tied financially to the HMO.

Many specialists also distrusted HMOs because they also detested the feeling of having to justify their decisions to, God forbid, a primary care doctor.

Adding to the problem, some HMOs were indeed greedy and corrupt and not interested in providing quality care. So, few in the healthcare industry wept when the era came to an untimely close and the United States health insurance industry went back to a fee-for-service environment.

Unfortunately, double-digit health inflation returned with a vengeance.

The lesson here is HMOs worked. They changed incentives and controlled costs. The movement died—with a notable few exceptions such as Kaiser Permanente—because of consumer and physician resistance.

The improvement in cost from that era was not lost on the Obama administration. The HMO concept found its way into this country's current reform legislation under the pseudonym Accountable Care Organizations.

Another element impacting the singularity of the doctor/patient relationship is the emergence of evidence-based medicine. In an earlier chapter, the importance of variation in the practice of medicine was noted. The art and science of medicine requires each physician to apply his or her unique blend of intuition and scientific knowledge to each patient's condition. This freedom, when applied to the lack of financial disincentives from overuse by both patients and physicians, leads to great variations in what services patients receive.

There are some standards and consistencies in how patients are treated that can reduce this variation. These protocols, often called evidence-based medicine, must be part of any plan that hopes to restrain those costs.

There are protocols delivered by leading medical schools that guide physicians down pathways for the most efficient and humane care of patients. By following the "evidence," variation, and thus cost, are reduced.

However, if we believe that care decisions are only between us and our doctors, we will miss the opportunity for the efficiencies that evidenced-based medicine will provide.

• The third cliché that limits our understanding and hinders any ability to have thoughtful discussions about health care is that the new legislation will provide health care to all Americans. What it may do is provide insurance coverage to all Americans. Coverage implies an individual has a source of payment for the medical services he or she may receive from the health system.

Coverage is far different than access. The term *access* means you can get an appointment to see a doctor. Access implies all the resources of the health system are available. It is likely millions of Americans will have coverage for the first time, but access still will be an issue. Across this country, millions of people hold a Medicaid card, a Federal/State program for certain elements of the poor. This guarantees them nothing in terms of access to doctors' offices.

Significant numbers of doctors simply refuse to see Medicaid patients, a silent protest of what many physicians see as extraordinarily low reimbursement for their services. Increasingly, many physicians are limiting the number of Medicare patients in their practice for exactly the same reason.

As a new reform package significantly increases the number of Medicaid recipients, would physicians react any differently as long as they have the option of filling their practice with commercially insured patients and thus receive higher reimbursement? History seems to indicate many doctors would continue to operate in their own best interest by refusing to see these newly-anointed Medicaid patients.

- There are two words that are the most destructive to having an adult conversation about health reform. This is the accusation that proponents of reform were engaged in creating *death panels*. This accusation inevitably led to an examination of the Medicare program. Any review of Medicare clearly exposes a program with explosive growth that threatens to bankrupt our economy.

  end of life care

  The fact is, our elderly are living far beyond expectations when the program started in 1965. Our life expectancy has increased, and our birth rate has declined, all creating enormous cost pressures on the Medicare program.

  Despite these obvious problems, the fact is the cost pressure is exacerbated by the enormous variation on how our elderly are treated across this country. This variation is unexplained and costly. We do complex treatments for Medicare patients when there are no improvements in life expectancy. Also not uncommon are complex surgeries involving general anesthesia for palliative reasons, and rigorous and debilitating chemotherapy with little chance of survival.

These decisions are often made for patient comfort and because there are little or no financial consequences for the patient or family. We routinely have conversations about heroic treatments and surgeries for our elderly that would never take place in the rest of the world. A conversation about what decisions make humane and economic sense would seem to be appropriate.

However, the words are barely out of one's mouth until the term *death panels* is applied. Intelligent debate then becomes impossible as both pro and con proponents retreat to their respective corners muttering the platitudes that make both feel good about themselves but shed little light on a difficult subject.

• The proponents of reform figured out quickly that selling reform on the basis of improved coverage for the poor was an interesting but not very compelling argument. They moved with lightning speed to change the argument from "coverage for all" to "insurance reform."

After all, everybody distrusts insurance companies. Who doesn't have a story about their auto, homeowners, or even their medical insurer acting badly, making what appears to be arbitrary, capricious, and self-serving decisions?

Making reform of medical insurance the lynch pin of the discussions was a master-stroke of political theatre.

The key tenet of insurance reform was the coverage of pre-existing conditions. An understandable fear of many people is the inability to get medical insurance after a diagnosis of some chronic disease. The problem of losing our job while a member of our family is being treated for cancer and then not being eligible for coverage with our new employer because of a preexisting condition is a very real and scary prospect.

So President Obama cleverly led the discussion with conversation about insurance reform. The primary focus here was the elimination of preexisting condition qualifiers.

The only problem from an insurance perspective, not a humane one, is that covering preexisting conditions makes absolutely no sense as an insurance concept. This requirement would ask an insurance carrier to cover a known risk.

The whole principle behind insurance is to take a premium, which is a bet, that the insurance company will cover your unknown risk and estimate their losses through underwriting against the total premium dollars they collect.

Covering known risks is a very bad bet for an insurance company. If my driving record is full of accidents, along with numerous DWIs, the chance of anyone insuring me without substantial penalties is very slim. My past behavior as a predictor of future behavior is clearly a known risk that becomes difficult, if not impossible, to insure.

This comparison is made for illustrative purposes. There is no fault for those unlucky enough to get cancer or to be in an accident. However, from the insurance company's perspective the economic result is the same.

To insure a known cancer patient simply means the insurer has already lost the bet. This is not insurance. It is a payment scheme. So it is not a surprise that as soon as reform passed with requirements on preexisting conditions, insuring children until age twenty-six, and eliminating lifetime reserves, the insurers immediately moved to hedge their bet by substantially raising premiums.

It was all too predictable.

• The final phrase that comes trippingly to the lips of proponents of the health reform plan is, "If you like your doctor and your health plan, you will be able to keep them." I am sorry. This is clearly disingenuous. The president and his followers routinely utter this phrase. Unfortunately, it does not jive with the thrust of their plan.

The destruction of employee-based insurance, resulting mainly in health insurance to be sold as an individual product, would drive us to a fracture of that traditional relationship. In essence, what is being said is that everything we understood about our physician and insurance relationship must change. But, by the way, nothing will change for you as an individual. It may be politically necessary to assuage our worst fears. However, it simply makes no sense given the logic of the legislation.

My belief is we must have a tough adult conversation about the financing and delivery of health services to ever get a plan that accomplishes the goal of covering the most people with consistent quality and affordable prices.

As long as we retreat to our television sound bites, such as, "we have the best health care system in the world," or, "health care decisions should only be between you and your doctor," or, "you can keep your doctor and insurance plan," then thoughtful debate becomes practically impossible. These sound bites take the place of any real intense examination of the issues.

Once politicians of all stripes retreat to these poll-tested phrases, any intellectual conversation is impossible. All they imply is the American public is not smart enough to take all the variables, alternatives, and consequences into account. The conversation ultimately falls back into our clichés because real, thoughtful debate simply is beyond our intellectual capacity or our willingness to consider other positions.

Patient Protection and Affordable Care Act: Important but Flawed Legislation

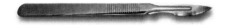

More good things can happen when you do not care who gets the credit.

—Benjamin Franklin

The Republicans should have seen it coming. The Democrats telegraphed their signals long before the 2010 debate and passage of health reform. The basis of what emerged was thoroughly discussed in Tom Daschle's book, *Critical: What We Can Do About the Health Care Crisis*, as well as Ezekiel Emanuel's *Health Care Guaranteed*.

It was all laid out. The employer mandate, the individual mandate, the exchanges, the elimination of employer-based insurance, and the oversight by a national panel of experts to review the appropriateness of medical interventions were all clearly delineated.

The Republicans had plenty of time to advance their own ideas on how to accomplish the goal, i.e. more coverage, higher quality, less cost. Unfortunately, even with all these warnings, they were still left at the starting gate muttering something about market-based solutions. The Republicans were portrayed as the Party of No—no ideas, no alternatives, no imaginative thinking.

The Democrats were just as obtuse. They were so committed to sticking to the game plan they failed to factor in the realization that 50 percent of the country was probably not ready for the comprehensiveness of their heartfelt desires. So both sides retreated to their ideological corners.

Health Cost Formula

Perhaps the first step in understanding health care reform legislation is to review the basic elements of how Americans pay for health care. This understanding can be summarized in a basic—albeit highly simplified—equation: \$=number of plan participants x structure of benefits x provider payments.

For simplicity's sake, I will summarize this as \$=PP1 x SB x PP2.

This formula tells us much of what we need to understand about the cost of health coverage. More specifically, we can identify how the ultimate price tag is altered by changing—up or down—any of the multipliers in this equation.

- First and most obvious, is the number of people covered. Employers who generally subsidize a major portion of their employees' health plan understand adding employees and their families only exacerbates their cost problem. Thus, the political commentators are correctly noting that expanded mandates for coverage only act as a depressor of job growth.

  The Medicare program is fractured simply by the number of senior citizens who are living substantially beyond the life expectancy predicted when the program started. Logic tells us that adding millions of new Americans with health coverage will require substantially more tax dollars unless one or both of the other two elements in the equation can be reduced.

- Structure of benefits essentially means what is covered in the health plan. Does the plan cover the basics such as emergency room visits and hospitalization, or is it more esoteric to cover areas such as preventative care, well baby care, or even cosmetic surgery?

  The broader the plan, obviously, the more costly the premium. We already have noted how required coverage for certain maladies becomes a political contest in every state legislature. No matter where the line is drawn in defining plan coverage, someone on the other side of that line will be enraged and lobby hard for mandated coverage of their disease. This ultimately raises the cost for everyone.

Structure of benefits also includes the whole concept of the individual's responsibility to pay for part of their care. The most obvious element is the size of the deductible. This is a basic insurance concept that made the jump from auto and home insurance into health care. In its most basic format, the deductible is a way for the insurance claimant to have skin in the game. Insurance recovery does not start until the deductible is satisfied. A deductible limits the insurance company's exposure to losses exceeding the deductible. It helps insurance companies assure it is only covering major losses.

Since the claimant must pay for losses up to the deductible limit before their insurance kicks in, the size of the deductible is inversely proportional to the premium. Raising the deductible lowers the premium. Thus, one sure way to control premium growth is for the insured to take even greater risk for their losses by accepting even larger deductibles.

When I started working in health care in 1970, the typical deductibles were in the $50 to $100 range. Today, a deductible of $1,000 or more is not uncommon. Beleaguered employers have long understood shifting more responsibility onto their employees lowers their annual health care costs.

The most costly employees to cover are those protected by a union contract that eliminates the employers' ability to raise deductibles. Low deductibles, and thus low barriers to entry into the health system, are directly tied to high utilization of the medical system.

We may, however, be reaching the outer limits of how high deductibles can be raised. A low-income earner with a $1,000 deductible for each member of his family is often for all intents and purposes uninsured. They simply cannot satisfy the deductible.

Co-payments serve the same purpose. By requiring patients to pay part of the cost of a physician's office visit, it forces individuals to consider whether they really need to see their doctor. Thus, the cost of health care for the individual, the employer, or even the government can be altered by changing both plan coverage and the individual's personal responsibility for paying part of the cost.

- The third multiplier in our equation is the payment to those individuals or entities who actually deliver care. This obviously includes doctors and hospitals. But there are a host of other health providers who also feed at the health care trough.

These include clinical labs, urgent care centers, pharmacies, home health providers, in-home equipment suppliers, hospices—the list goes on. Each of these entities tries desperately to raise their reimbursement from the payers.

Hospitals routinely negotiate with insurance companies. The companies, using the size of their pool of insureds as leverage, attempt to provide as little reimbursement as the providers will accept.

Large hospital systems or hospitals with great reputations—an M.D. Anderson, for instance—use their size or their stellar reputation to maximize the payment schedule they receive from the insurance companies. If negotiations break down, the insurance company may find it difficult to sell their product without that hospital or system as part of their covered provider network.

An employer's worst fear is to contract for employee health coverage and have their employees disappointed by not finding their favorite doctor or hospital on the list of covered providers. Good hospitals understand this fear and use it vigorously to press for higher reimbursement.

Both sides of this negotiation fully realize the high stakes game being played. Insurers effectively use the size of their provider network to stimulate the hospital and other providers to deeply discount the price for their services. The insurers trade a smaller network for deeper discounts from the providers. The hospital knows a smaller network of their competitors means more patients will find their way to their hospital services.[1]

With more of their costs covered, the hospitals can afford to give the carrier deeper discounts. It is volume discounting, pure and simple. This volume discounting is what Walmart does every day. They know if they buy a million units of a product, they can demand a better price than if they buy far fewer. For a hospital, fewer competitors in a network mean more patients. So the hospitals trade volume for price.

Recall the analogy of my daughter shopping with my credit card. In this case, the price for a dress using my MasterCard may be different than someone else purchasing a dress using a Visa. This is a thumbnail version of pricing in health care. Since price negotiations are highly individualized to each carrier and since government programs set their own reimbursement levels, the ultimate price may vary widely.

Parenthetically, this practice leads to one of the great misunderstandings in paying for health care. The allegation is often made that a private patient pays more than an insured patient for the same service. This is technically correct. However, most hospitals will make allowances for some private discounting of the bill based on the patient's income. This includes totally free services for the poorest among us.

Thus, the point is, controlling health costs is mathematically very simple. One or more of the multipliers must be reduced while holding the others reasonably constant. While the arithmetic is easy, reducing any of the elements proves very tricky.

Simple Logic

Here is the logic.

If the desire is to cover more people in reform legislation, then either the benefit structure or provider payments must be reduced. Politically, the latter is significantly more palatable. The public might care less what doctors and hospitals get paid. However, every action has a reaction.

The unintended consequences of reduced physician payments for Medicaid means thousands of doctors simply refuse to see patients with that coverage. Remember here the difference between access and coverage. Low reimbursement for provider payments could surely bring some already distressed hospitals to their knees.

Some Americans might consider this a good thing, but an unintended consequence could be that hospitals in our most distressed urban and rural areas might be the first to be impacted. Continued low payments also would force the closure of many financially marginal hospital programs, such as a neighborhood free clinic, in favor of more profitable services.

While cutting provider payments is surely in the future for doctors and hospitals, there is simply not enough money in a scorched earth policy to totally offset the cost of the increase of all the new entrants into health coverage.

That leaves us only one alternative.

In order to cover more people and hold cost constant, we must tackle what the new coverage will finance and how much of a personal responsibility each of us will have.

In the first part of this book, we discussed if health care *is* a right, then that right *must* be defined. By definition, that means we must be clear about to what each of us is entitled simply by virtue of being an American. Again, if cost control is as important as expanding coverage, then the reasonable conclusion is that both the benefits and what we as individuals must pay is a difficult but necessary condition for meeting that goal.

During the debate over health reform in 2010, the concept of what benefits should be included was acidulously avoided and ultimately left to the Secretary of Health and Human Services to determine. Rightly so; it is a no-win discussion politically for either side. It was so difficult even the president's closest allies did not dare venture into that minefield.

In fact, the only time a political body was bold enough to attempt an intelligent debate on benefit structure was in the 1990s in the Oregon Legislature. Led by Governor John Kitzhaber, Oregon did something unprecedented. They clearly saw if they wanted to cover more people in the Medicaid program and hold their health budget constant, then what was covered must be reduced.

In most state legislatures during budget-crunch time, in order to keep Medicaid costs in control, the number of covered people is reduced. The minimum income level for eligibility is lowered, and thus, thousands suddenly become too rich to qualify for Medicaid. Oregon's clever idea was to use reverse engineering. Rather than controlling costs by tossing people off the Medicaid rolls, they moved to cover as many people as possible and limit what was covered. They understood the equation, $\$=PP1 \times SB \times PP2$.

Oregon's technique for choosing what to cover was equally clever. Through an open public discussion, they rank ordered, for their societal and individual value, all the possible services for which Medicaid might pay. Then, they calculated given average-use rates, what each service would cost the state's Medicaid program. These costs were added together, and when they reached the state's existing budget for Medicaid, they simply drew a line. The state would cover anything below the line and nothing above the line. As a result, their philosophy of maintaining the budget—not by cutting people off the rolls but by cutting what they would reimburse—was promulgated.

Sadly, this grand adventure did not survive as a model for national use as it should have. Citizens and interested groups on the other side of the line exercised their political muscle and began to move that line covering more services until the brilliant plan was essentially neutered. After discussing the factors that make American health care different, ideological statements that make intelligent discussion difficult, some basic rules of insurance, and finally health care arithmetic, we should review the health care reform plan that emerged.

The attempt here is not an exhaustive review of the legislation but an effort to explain the logic behind the plan. Clearly, some readers will argue with that logic. The challenge here is not to justify it but to simply understand its overarching concepts.

The "Act"

The *Patient Protection and Affordable Care Act* leads in its very first section with the idea of insurance reforms, placed up front to specifically draw attention to the most popular part of the legislation.

The centerpiece of the bill, if we are to believe its promoters, is insurance reform. The implication here is that certain requirements must be included in insurance policy offerings because these companies are simply too greedy to offer these consumer-friendly alternatives on their own.

The key to the requirement is to cover preexisting conditions. This addresses the average American's greatest fear: being without coverage at their most vulnerable time when a major chronic disease hits.

Other sweeteners were added covering dependent children until age twenty-six and the elimination of lifetime reserves. The former answers the question of this generation of young adults who are struggling to find work but in the end must depend on their parents for support. The latter insures those with prolonged health issues will never run out of coverage. These are clearly consumer-friendly additions, specially designed to curry favor among the electorate.

Unfortunately, the drafters of this legislation paid little attention to the basic principles of insurance or to our equation of health care costs. If they had been logical and not political, they would have understood there was no way to place additional requirements on health insurers and hold premiums constant.

Like all additional benefits, these goodies come at a price. The immediate reaction of the insurance market was to cover their bets and raise premiums. This was the first of several questionable assumptions built into the legislation. The assumption was that this legislation would not produce substantial premium increases.

However, the insurance companies moved swiftly to protect their margins and massively raised premiums in anticipation of these new requirements.

The second major thrust of this legislation was the establishment of state insurance exchanges. This was envisioned as an Internet marketplace for individuals. Many of the newly covered would use the exchange to make decisions about what policies meet their individual needs. The states could add benefits to the basic package but must pay for them. They also must establish toll-free lines and Internet websites, develop standard plan formats, and certify plans for inclusion in the list of consumer options.

Although these state exchanges will be highly regulated, it could be argued they are the ultimate free market device. Individuals will make decisions concerning their insurance choices based on a plethora of information presented in a standard format. We will, in essence, be buying health insurance at the kitchen table. The employer will not be making the decision for us. What could be more free market driven?

Mandates

Why will the employer not be making these choices for us? It is called the *employer mandate*. In its simplest form, every employer will be required to furnish a "standard policy" that meets minimum requirements for their employees or pay a fee.

Here will be the thought process for the employer: *I can continue to provide health insurance for my employees, take the risk for premium increases, and continue to deal with a human resources headache, or I can pay a penalty fee and send my employees to the exchange.*

This is a no-brainer.

Most employers who provide health insurance do so simply because they cannot compete for talent without it. Once everyone is covered, the playing field is level. Why not pay the fee? It is the same money without the irritation.

Hence, in a relatively short period, most employers will move their employees into the exchange, and employer-based insurance as we know it will be only a distant memory.

The most controversial part of the health reform plan is the individual mandate. This provision specifies that each of us must maintain minimum health care coverage or pay a penalty. The idea deeply offends conservatives who find it outrageous, and perhaps unconstitutional, to force an individual to buy a product they may not want.

Setting aside the constitutional argument for a moment, the mandate does have its own logic. Generally, those most desiring health insurance are those who need it the most.

Covering preexisting conditions, for instance, is a very bad deal for insurers unless their risk is spread over a very wide population. Only by covering a large pool of insureds can the insurer's risk be mitigated. Thus, the requirement for all of us to play in the insurance game makes perfect sense if the goal is to require insurers to do something that makes no economic sense.

There is also the responsibility argument. A man exceeding the speed limit on a motorcycle, smoking a cigarette, and not wearing a helmet passed me on the freeway. While this is the height of a lack of personal responsibility, my first thought was, *I bet he has no health insurance.*

If I was correct and he became a head injury case in the emergency room, then all of us with insurance would finance his care, as hospitals shift the cost of this ne'er-do-well to those of us with health insurance. The argument for an individual mandate is that some of us simply must be required to do the right thing.

Every state requires we have auto insurance before we drive a car. While enforcement varies from state to state, the mandate that we buy something is constant. Have you ever talked to an insured motorist who has had an accident with an uninsured driver? The outrage is palpable.

I suspect many of those most upset with the individual mandate are somehow very comfortable with the mandate that all those other drivers out there also should have auto insurance.

This analogy is limited in its application. Auto insurance is a state mandate that has far fewer implications for each of us than health insurance, but it is a perfect example of a government requirement for us to buy a product that we might otherwise choose not to purchase.

The other issue with the mandate is the size of the penalty the individual must pay. If it's too low, citizens will simply gamble on the need for health coverage. As we found in Massachusetts with their individual mandate, individuals would calculate their risk of needing insurance and simply pay the fee until the likelihood of their needing health insurance became evident. Then, they would jump back into the system for a brief period of time. This gaming of the system is a consequence of a fee that does not act as a disincentive to abuse.

The subject of mandates ~ both employer and individual ~ is clearly the most controversial piece of the legislation. If left unchanged by court action it will have the most profound impact on how insurance is provided and acquired in this country.

Expanding Medicaid

Currently, there are roughly thirty-two million uncovered Americans. Half of these will gain coverage in this legislation by expanding Medicaid.

Medicaid started in 1965 as companion legislation to Medicare. The latter was a totally federal program to provide coverage to all of those over sixty-five. Medicaid was far narrower. The threshold to get into Medicare was just to live until sixty-five. Medicaid was basically a program that declared that some poor people and some diseases were more important than others.

If you were a poor woman or disabled or you had breast or cervical cancer, you could get coverage. If you were a poor young male or had the misfortune to have some other kind of cancer, sorry. Fend for yourself. The right disease, the right age, the right sex, then come on down; you are qualified.

In addition, since Medicaid is partially funded by the state and administered by them, the level of income needed to qualify varies widely by state. With the *Patient Protection and Affordable Care Act*, there will be a uniform national threshold of 133 percent of poverty, roughly $14,000 per year for individuals. All other categories disappear. The newly eligible will be 100 percent financed by the federal government, ultimately trailing off to 90 percent financing beyond the year 2020.

Public Option

The most controversial piece of reform legislation that failed to make it through the arduous political process was the infamous government or public option.

A public option was conceived as one choice an individual could make in choosing a plan from the state exchange. Here the federal government could offer through the exchange a competitive product (perhaps similar to Medicare) to those offered by private insurance companies. This proposal was very dear to the president's most arduous supporters. They vigorously argued this was the best way to keep honest those competing insurance companies authorized to do business in the exchange.

This claim, perhaps a bit disingenuously, was that public option would be the essence of a free market. Their logic was that those searching the exchange would have the ability to simply compare the insurer's product with that of a government-issued policy.

Their opponents logically stated the government would have a significant advantage in this competition. While insurance companies must negotiate with providers over the pricing of services, the government could simply mandate what it would pay. The capability of dictating what it will pay for provider services, which is exactly what happens in Medicare, gives it leverage unmatched by insurance carriers.

The analogy here would be for a grocery store's largest customer to note they were willing to buy their produce, but they were not willing to pay the grocery store's stated prices. Instead, they will only pay 50 percent of the grocer's cost and, oh, by the way, the grocer would be required to sell it at that discount. That buyer could then sell that produce at a fraction of the cost of another buyer paying the grocer's full price.

This is essentially how our Medicare program works. The provider community makes available its service at a fraction of its cost to governmental patients simply because it has no other choice. So it should be little wonder the insurance industry and provider groups resisted the public option.

Reform opponents correctly anticipated this discount advantage. They foresaw, I believe with accuracy, that the insurance companies would be at such a competitive disadvantage, their ability to sell a product would be quickly eliminated. As one by one the carriers left this prejudiced market, we would ultimately be left with only the government option.

Provider groups were threatened because only on their privately insured patients can they create any margin. If patients move quickly to a public option, their favorable pricing from insurance carriers would quickly disappear.

Thus, by de facto, we would emerge into a single-payer system. By default, we would get what the reformers really wanted all along and what the conservatives fear the most: a single-payer system. As it turns out, because of this resistance, the president eventually had to trade the public option for votes.

Outcomes Research

A second controversial piece that also landed on the cutting room floor was the creation of a national agency that would make decisions about which treatments and therapies deserve recognition and reimbursement.

New technology routinely enters the market, often only marginally better than existing technology. Evidence to support this generally more expensive therapy or diagnostic tool is frequently sketchy. The proponents of this new technology—such as device manufacturers, physicians who may have a vested interest in the project, hospitals looking for a competitive advantage—all have sizeable vested interest.

These interest groups all promote enhanced reimbursement from the payers, sometimes based on little clinical evidence of its superiority over existing technology.

This idea mentioned in Senator Daschle's book was the creation of an impartial agency staffed by board members with impeccable scientific credentials and not tied to any vested interest. This group would then make presumably informed and dispassionate judgments about new therapies and diagnostic tools.

The model here is the Federal Reserve Board, able to make far-reaching decisions on complex issues, unencumbered by political ties or vicissitudes of a fickle market place.

The legislation, however, comes close to this concept in its call for a "Patient-Centered Outcomes Research Institute," a public-private board appointed by the U.S. Comptroller General to provide outcomes research. The concept would be to develop research that would answer the question, "What really works in medicine?"

But true to the political nature of the legislation, the research of this institute must be politically correct. As a tip of the hat to the "care should only be between you and your physician" crowd, this institute is prohibited from any findings that could be construed as "practice guidelines."

Physician specialty societies and some medical schools have developed protocols to address how patients with similar symptoms should be diagnosed and treated. These guidelines are often framed on the basis of what some termed "evidence-based medicine." Other physicians call the guidelines "cook-book medicine." We will attempt later to make the case that following the evidence is the best way to begin to control medical costs.

As we will see, this is a mistake. If we are to accomplish the goal of covering more people while keeping quality and cost relatively constant, we will require a move to evidenced-based medicine, as discussed in chapter two.

There are a number of other interesting parts of this legislation that deserve at least a passing nod.

1. There are limitations on deductibles required: $2,000 for individuals and $4,000 for families.

2. There are requirements for the Secretary of Health and Human Services to establish criteria for qualified plans to be included in the state exchanges. Thus, the federal government will set the ground rules for participation in the exchange.

3. There are requirements for insurers to pool the risk for all enrollees of an offered plan, regardless of whether the plan is offered in the exchange or not.

    This deserves a note. In the early days of health insurance, underwriting was done on a community-rated basis. In other words, the risk for all covered employees from all companies was treated the same. As insurance became more competitive, insurers began offering company-rated plans. This allowed those companies with younger and fewer female employees a lower-risk profile and, thus, lower premiums.

    Younger males are shown to have far fewer encounters with the health system than their older and female counterparts. The result of company-rated plans was to disadvantage companies with these population groups. Presumably, this pooling of risk could now raise premiums for employers with demographics of younger and male employees, and lower premiums for employers with predominantly older and female workers.

The legislation stimulates and rewards the formation of Accountable Care Organizations (ACOs) for Medicare patients. These ACOs get to keep a percentage of the savings they might generate. Think of them as Health Maintenance Organizations (HMOs) revisited.

4. The legislation provides programs for bundling of payments. The idea here is to begin paying a flat fee for all services surrounding an individual patient encounter with the health system. In other words, one payment for all hospital, physician, and post-hospital services surrounding an admission to the hospital.

5. The legislation calls for a requirement for drug manufacturers to provide a 50-percent discount to all Part D Medicare beneficiaries.

6. The legislation provides for coverage with no deductibles for Medicare patients who receive wellness visits.

7. The legislation provides forcoverage with no deductibles for Medicaid patients who get tobacco cessation services.

8. The legislation stipulates that chain restaurants with twenty or more locations will be required to disclose calorie counts on all menu items.

9. The legislation provides for significant grants and incentives to promote the education of more primary care physicians.

10. The legislation limits physician-owned hospitals from participating in Medicare if they had no provider agreement prior to February 2010. This effectively limits future physician-owned hospitals. This, of course, does not touch physician ownership of the myriad other outpatient services currently owned by doctors.

11. The legislation makes a very weak reference to the medical malpractice issue. There is an encouragement to the states to develop alternatives to civil litigation. This is a rather pathetic nod to a significant problem.

12. The legislation mandates a list of fees on device manufacturers, pharmaceutical companies, and insurance companies to help finance this package.

This is only a small handful of the thousands of pages, features, and requirements in this massive bill. The underlying principles, such as the exchanges and the mandates, are the real intellectual underpinnings of the legislation and consequently deserve the most attention.

I hope by now my central thesis has become clear. We have been ill served by both sides of the political spectrum. The president and his Democratic allies in Congress were disingenuous when they insisted, "If you like your insurance carrier, you can keep it." They were either deluding themselves and us, or they simply had not thought through the intellectual implications of what they were proposing.

The Democratic leadership in Congress was obviously so intent on bringing this legislation to reality, it really did stretch the bounds or reasonableness in how the legislation would be financed. As a consequence, what could have been a laudable effort essentially was converted into smoke and mirrors to make the numbers work.

There are at least three areas of dubious arithmetic.

First, the assumption was made the plan would be paid for in part by future Medicare reform cost savings. So we are to believe our spineless Congress, at some point in the future, will actually cut benefits, raise taxes, or have an income test for Medicare. There is nothing in their history to suggest they are up to the task.

Barring a debacle such as we recently saw in Greece, this isn't going to happen. The Greeks, who are on the edge of financial insolvency, have found it virtually impossible to take away benefits its public has come to expect.

Second, very costly fixes were conveniently left out of the bill. The most obvious is the so-called "doctors' fix." For the past several years, every few months, Congress has been forced to delay a huge cut in doctors' fees that were programmed by former legislation to have already taken place. The permanent fix for this problem—$250 billion to $300 billion—was never counted in the cost of health reform.

Third, the bill anticipates future revenue by taxing so-called "Cadillac" plans. It is true, some high-paid executives have richer plans than their employees, but many union plans also fall into this category. Again, are we to believe some future Congress is really up to the challenge of taxing health plans that historically have been provided as a tax-free benefit?

The Republicans were just as guilty. Every discussion about any change was met with poll-tested incendiary bombs such as "death panels."

As a consequence, this highly charged and highly partisan debate over the *Patient Protection and Affordable Care Act* was a tragically lost opportunity to make a real difference for the American public.

A pox on both their houses.

Common-Sense Solutions

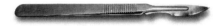

> Every morning in Africa a gazelle wakes up knowing that if he cannot outrun the fastest lion, he will be eaten. That same morning the lion wakes up and knows that if she cannot outrun the slowest gazelle, she will starve.
>
> —African Proverb

Perspective is everything. My perspective on health reform is certainly not gospel, just my opinion, but an opinion informed by almost forty years as a hospital CEO. It is a perspective made more credible by conversations with many smart people. Physicians, nurses, insurance executives, vendors, health educators, and hospital executives, as well as many friends and neighbors, have helped me shape these recommendations.

This next section is, indeed, the hard part. We have taken an extensive look at our unique American health system. In doing so, we speculated any changes to that system must, at the very least, acknowledge this uniqueness and, if not address it totally, at least allow for its impact and the resistance to change it is likely to generate.

We have examined politics of highly charged rhetoric, which influences every debate. We reviewed the intellectual underpinnings of the *Patient Protection and Affordable Care Act*, or as its opponents derisively call it, "Obamacare."

So the moment of truth has arrived and, as my wife might say, "Okay, Mr. Smarty Pants, what would you do?" This chapter is not a blueprint for comprehensive reform. It is meant to simply stimulate critical thinking around a complex problem. The concepts are straightforward. They are meant only as building blocks on which a comprehensive reform package could be constructed.

I have a distinct advantage. I am not running for political office. I must please no one. My observations and recommendations are based on a simple point of view.

Both sides of the political spectrum have it right some of the time and wrong most of the time. The problem is we have let the politicians lead the debate. On the most critical decision of this generation, we have let the least knowledgeable among us dictate the limits of our thought process.

In the absence of a national debate around such explosive issues as care of the elderly, we have substituted the rantings of politicians with suspect motives. This is a group that, with few exceptions, has never cared for a patient, never developed a medical service, and often, never even met a payroll.

This group's only connection to the health system has been as a patient or, perhaps, as the family of a patient.

For many of these people who are now making decisions concerning the most important domestic issue of our time, they have been protected by the richest health benefit plan in America. Members of Congress simply have it better than the rest of us.

So I humbly present my perspective. The question I have continually asked those with whom I have consulted is, "If you were king and could devise a health care system that covered more people, maintained or even improved quality, and constrained cost, what would you do?"

Thus, we start with an admittedly prejudiced position. That is, our first goal is to cover more people. Expanding coverage is lost in the acrimonious debate about repealing health care legislation. Is this really still the ultimate goal?

At one time, I thought the goal was clear. Covering the uninsured was the principle motivation. The idea that one-fourth to one-third of our population had no health insurance coverage was universally accepted as a blight on our national character. Above all else, this problem must be solved.

Current rhetoric might lead us to believe this goal has somehow disappeared. Supporters of this legislation almost never mention coverage of the uninsured as an overarching motivator. What we hear instead are conversations about insurance reform, tax credits for small businesses, or free wellness exams.

Debate over coverage for our most at-risk citizens has all but disappeared from the public stage. It is as if this issue had no political traction. Despite its disappearance from the conversation, my purpose here is to resurrect it as a principle goal in health reform.

Given my prejudice, the logic of these presented solutions becomes relatively straightforward. Our simple equation from the previous chapter—$\$=PP1 \times SB \times PP2$—tells us that if our goal is to add more people as insured, then we must find a way to reduce or control the other variables. This is necessary in order to not bankrupt the country with a new insurance entitlement.

Let me put a personal face on this population. Lucy is a regular at a free clinic our organization has run for several years in one of the most distressed areas of Oklahoma City. She is a single mother of two. Lucy works two jobs. One of her jobs is as a domestic; the other is in a fast-food restaurant. Neither of these jobs provides Lucy health insurance.

Lucy's income is approximately $12,000 a year. This makes her too rich to qualify for Medicaid. So our clinic becomes the medical home for her and her children.

Lucy pays property and sales taxes and perhaps some state and federal income tax. She is a contributing member to our community. To my mind, she is exactly the kind of individual for whom we started this journey. Unfortunately, we have lost our focus on Lucy and her children.

It is certainly true a number of the uninsured are those with the ability to buy insurance but who simply choose not to. Our cyclist riding around without a helmet while smoking may well be one of these. While I have little sympathy for this gentleman, this is exactly the kind of person to whom the individual mandate was aimed.

This guy games the system. He knows the rest of us will finance his care when he crashes his motorcycle and shows up in a hospital emergency room. We condone and support his irresponsibility as he thumbs his nose at the rest of us in the name of individual choice.

The needs of both Lucy and the cyclist must be addressed in our proposed system.

The first thing that must be done is to stop!

Stop the implementation of health care reform.

Stop the efforts to repeal it.

Stop all political rhetoric on both sides.

Call a halt to discussions of the issues in Congress.

We are simply not ready to let our most prejudiced politicians control and dominate the proceedings. Before we toss them the ball, we need at least a year of thoughtful, serious, and adult discussions aimed at letting our citizens have the opportunity to listen, think, study, observe, and speak to the complex issues facing us.

My premise, for instance, is we cannot solve the Medicare problem unless we patiently listen to each other debate appropriate care for our elderly. We cannot address the costly variation in health care unless we allow the experts to explain the reasoning behind evidenced-based medicine. We need to hear our best physicians explain the dangers, as well as the upside, of following the evidence.

We must educate ourselves about the frustrations of our physicians who attempt to practice good medicine but often are sabotaged by their own patients' demands for unhealthy or unneeded treatments, diagnostic tests, or medications.

The perfect example is the pressure patients put on physicians to order costly antibiotics to fight viral infections. Most of our winter flus are caused by viruses rather than bacteria. Antibiotics, which fight bacteria, are ineffective to treat viral infections.

These discussions would be to inform, not critique, other positions. Many people do not have a clue on the inner workings of this country's health system. These same people, however, may be willing to take to the streets, impassioned by the proponents of a particular political position.

My idea here is to have these discussions sponsored by a combination of public and private dollars. These discussions would be conducted by nonpartisan, respected organizations, such as the American Heart Association or other national foundations involved in health care.

No organization tied directly or indirectly to a specific political party or philosophy should conduct these sessions. No politicians would be allowed to speak. The media would be invited to cover the discussions, but not to participate.

Imagine how threatening this would be to the politicians and to the cable news. They would not be allowed to tell us what we should think. In these public discussions, physicians could address the real world problems of delivering medical care. Health economists could speak to the financing of health care. Ethicists could hold forth on the ethics of our most intractable problems.

The best part would be an open dialogue and questions. No signs would be allowed. Civility would be strictly enforced. These discussions would close with participants making electronic choices of what they might do, given several painful but necessary alternatives as decision points.

If conducted correctly, the United States actually might have an opportunity to raise the understanding of the complexity of the issues involved. At the very least, we would be better-informed citizens and not be easily stampeded by either side. Only after a year of this do we give the ball back to the politicians.

This plan for a public debate strikes me as a brilliant idea. But to be historically honest, it has been tried before. The United States Medicare Prescription Drug Improvement and Modernization Act of 2003 required a public conversation very similar to the one I am suggesting.

In fifteen months, during 2005 and 2006, the Citizens' Health Care Working Group conducted a series of discussions across the United States to engage and challenge the public to debate and make choices concerning the shape of a future health care system. The group, appointed by the U.S. Comptroller General, made a concerted effort to answer four questions.

- What health care benefits and services should be provided?

- How does the American public want health care delivered?

- How should health care coverage be financed?

- What trade-offs are the American public willing to make in either benefits or financing to ensure access to affordable, high-quality health care coverage and services?

In 2006, the Working Groups' recommendations were delivered to the Secretary of Health and Human services and, apparently, died a very quiet death. These recommendations were thoughtful and diverse and deserved significantly more discussion. They would have served as a good framework for the 2010 Congressional debate. Many of the themes I will suggest reflect thinking similar to their efforts.

Why would my suggestion for a public debate be any different or meet a different end?

I believe there are two reasons.

First, the timing is altogether different. The United States now has reform legislation passed that has engendered great passion on both sides. That level of interest and enthusiasm did not exist in 2006. The same debate held today would have an intensity of coverage that was totally missing in 2006.

Second, in my concept, this debate should not be conducted by any branch of the government with the natural suspicion the results would be tilted by the influences of the current administration. In any case, the Working Group's report makes interesting reading.

I am convinced perverse incentives in our health care system got us into this mess.

Correct incentives could get us out. If we had set out fifty years ago to devise a system guaranteed to give us high cost and poor coverage, we have been remarkably successful.

Perverse Incentives

Let's review these incentives.

Physicians are rewarded on a production basis. The more they do, the more they get paid. Primary care physicians' financial incentives are to move patients rapidly through their offices at an accelerated pace.

Specialists are only rewarded when they perform their specialty. There is no incentive to move patients to the lowest level of care consistent with their individual needs. In fact, just the opposite is true. Their incentive is to move patients to the highest level of care and into the most expensive technology.

Karen Davis, president of the Commonwealth Fund, a respected think tank, notes, "Fee-for-service creates incentives for more and more services, even when there may be a lower cost way to treat a condition." It appears fee-for-service simply favors quantity over quality.

Similarly, hospitals' incentive is to maximize the number of patients in their facility and the use of high technology. The worst mix of patients for a hospital is a higher percentage of medical patients rather than surgical. Hospitals produce their best margin with patients receiving surgery and a significant number of high-cost diagnostic services. A patient sick in a bed with mostly nursing care as their major service component is a loser financially.

The hospital has no incentive to cooperate with its competitors on initiatives that might serve the public good.

There is no incentive to focus on public health problems. Hospital executives are highly motivated to get more and better technology than their competitors. They are incentivized to duplicate high-cost programs, such as cardiology, because of the favorable revenue it produces.

The fact these programs may already be provided elsewhere in their community is irrelevant to how the hospitals are rewarded.

The insurance carrier's incentives are also perverse. Since most are for-profit stock companies, their first loyalty is to their shareholders. As I noted in the chapter "What Makes American Health Care Unique," there is actually little classic insurance in what they do. The carriers are taking what is, in essence, a payment mechanism—taking money from one party and passing it to another while they take a cut in the process—and making it into a very good business.

Perhaps the most devastating consequence to this business model is their inability to think or care about the long-term consequences of their actions. Insurance carriers know from history their coverage of any particular company or individual is likely to be short term.

This is perhaps why they have been resistant to encouraging preventive health services. Since the payoff in healthier employees is sometime in the future, more than likely, some future carrier will reap the ultimate benefit. The insurance carriers get the up-front cost and are not around to get the reward from the lower cost of a healthier population. This focus on short-term rewards drives their inability to take a leadership role seriously in improving overall health of their enrollees.

Their incentive is also to delay as much as possible paying providers because of the enormous float of their investments. Their financial benefit is related to the time they can hang on to the provider's money. As a consequence, each carrier has its own forms, rules, and requirements.

This maze is difficult to manage and requires every provider to endure massive expense just to collect their bills. This complicated maze is singular to the American health system and adds 15 to 20 percent in cost to our health bill. *The Bloomberg Report* flatly states, "Patients are not the real customer, insurance companies are."

Americans, as patients, also have incentives that impact our ability to piece together a comprehensive and effective national health plan. Unfortunately, we have very little incentive to take care of ourselves. Public health initiatives (clean water, vaccinations) have added years to life expectancy.

Americans' behavior, however, accelerates the growth of chronic disease as the leading cause of death. We eat too much, consume too much alcohol, smoke excessively, and drive dangerously. Thus, heart disease, lung cancer, alcoholism, and traffic accidents are leading causes of death and disability, replacing infectious diseases our public health system has helped eliminate.

The fact is, we apparently have little incentive to improve our behavior. Just like our helmet-less motorcyclist, someone else will pay for the consequences of our bad behavior.

Who among us doesn't know of the hazards of smoking, yet millions of Americans light up every day?

Why?

My belief is there is in all of us a small amount of denial that misfortune will ever befall us. Our environment is also complicit in our self-deception. Our own schools feed our children the fattiest foods in school cafeterias and insure we have access to the highest caloric snacks and drinks in vending machines.

Cigarette manufacturers aim their advertising at the youngest and most vulnerable among us. Thus thousands of teenagers are addicted, condemning them to a lifetime of tobacco-related diseases.

Interestingly enough, our insurance system treats all of us the same. The smoker, the obese person, and the reckless driver pay the same premium as the individual who watches his or her weight, doesn't smoke, and drives safely.

Employers know their employees who smoke or who are significantly overweight are more expensive employees. Statistically they get sick more often, they take longer to recover, and they miss work more often.

Employer premiums are driven by the 80/20 rule: 20 percent of employees are responsible for 80 percent of the cost of health premiums for the group. This 20 percent tends to include those employees with the unhealthiest behaviors.

The obvious question is, why should employees who try their best to maintain their health be penalized with higher premiums by the 20 percent who appear determined to do damage to their bodies?

Today, many employers are moving to incentivize workers who meet certain health standards with lower premiums for their health insurance. Current law, however, limits how aggressive an employer can be in discriminating among employees based on health status. Congress should be encouraging these incentive programs, not limiting them.

In this litany of perverse incentives, we have not touched on the pharmaceutical industry or the device manufacturers or the many others whose ultimate desire is to maintain the status quo.

We started this book by pointing out our system would be very resistive to change. As we staggered through the 2010 debate over health reform, we got a small sample of just how entrenched these vested interests would be.

One side tells the American public the problem is that the health care reform legislation does nothing to control costs, while adding millions of newly insured. Their charge is that the legislation simply adds a new entitlement that ultimately will help bankrupt the country. This argument has merit.

Their opponents point out that, for the first time, insurance companies will not be able to abuse patients. They stress that state exchanges will be the ultimate marketplace. They also tout particular consumer-friendly parts of the legislation, such as the availability of wellness exams for the elderly.

This argument also has merit, but both sides are talking past each other. They both have missed the point.

The United States cannot cover millions more Americans and control costs without real, substantial change that will be difficult and, perhaps, painful.

A definition sometimes attributed to Albert Einstein and others is appropriate here: "Insanity: doing the same thing over and over again and expecting different results."

Thus, true to our original premise, our solution should and must be a mixture of free market and, yes, mandates when the market itself will not get us there.

First, we must have a public debate and discussion to educate our population and to prepare them for the difficult choices ahead of us.

Second, we must change the incentives now present in each part of the health system.

Changing Incentives

Insurers

Let's start with the insurance industry. If I am correct, and we have taken what in essence is a payment mechanism and tried to pretend it is true insurance, this would be a good place to start.

Our health system has taken an essentially claims processing function and allowed it to consume, under the heading of insurance, 20 percent of every health care dollar.

While not impugning the motives of health insurance executives, I believe, as an industry, they are trapped in an incentive process that not only allows but encourages them to act in a way counter to forming an effective American health system.

Thus, I propose we return to the insurance company's primary reason to exist—paying claims—and doing this rapidly and fairly. Their focus should be devoted primarily to receiving claims submitted by providers, comparing those claims to the benefit structure, and quickly dispatching payment.

This function has nothing to do with rewarding stockholders and advancing stock portfolios. Thus, these insurance companies should be not-for-profit. The reward system should be based on how quickly they can receive a claim, process it, and pay the appropriate amounts.

I do not believe in a single-payer system. I believe in a competitive industry motivated to excel in paying claims. Payers should have no incentive to make the claims processing as complicated as possible. Payment should be guaranteed to be processed quickly, if basic conditions are met. Providers could then reduce their overhead, now absorbed by huge collection staffs.

These new insurance companies would have to meet standards on claims processing speed. Once met and sustained, they could add a per-member, per-month fee to their cost base.

There are two other basic functions insurers are now performing. They negotiate with providers over fees, and those negotiations determine the size of their provider networks. I would propose they continue these functions. Since many Americans will now buy insurance over the Internet exchange, price sensitivity and network coverage become the determining factors that will drive their negotiations with providers.

We have noted that the benefits covered in any plan are a variable that impacts the overall cost of that plan. Benefit design was designated as "SB" in our formula. Obviously the richness of the benefit package will influence the ultimate cost of the plan.

Presumably, individual consumers working through the state exchanges will be able to design a plan that meets their individual needs. If the exchanges are designed correctly, the consumer should be able to connect their choices of benefits to their ultimate out-of-pocket costs.

For the first time, individuals will see a direct link between their choices and preferences and the ultimate premium consequences.

How do we move to a not-for-profit industry?

The free market should do it.

The new legislation already requires 80 percent of the insurer's cost to be in medical payments. Historically, insurers have called this percentage their *medical loss ratio*. That term alone tells us something about their business model. The primary purpose of insurers is to pay the benefits their members deserve; this function is inexplicably regarded as "loss."

The full intent is to keep this "loss" as small as possible. This new requirement would leave insurers with 20 percent of revenue to pay overhead, marketing, and profit.

In order to gain access to the exchange, insurers would have to agree to requirements on their speed of claims adjudication. With a medical loss ratio of 80 percent and specific requirements for speed of payments, the kinds of margins historically enjoyed will be hard to maintain. Capital, as it always does, will move to more lucrative opportunities.

A special Internal Revenue Service provision for insurance not-for-profits would be necessary. These entities—perhaps run as cooperatives by various industry groups—could emerge as a principle source of claims payment.

A classic niche market might result for those traditional for-profit insurers who might wish to maintain their margin and appeal to a slice of the American public intent on paying higher prices for exclusivity.

Reading between the lines of both United States Senator Tom Daschle's and Ezekiel Emanuel's books, the clear effort through a public option is to make health insurance as unprofitable as possible. As a result, insurers would eventually quit the market. In their minds, this would pave the way for a single-payer or government system.

This should not happen.

Changing the claims processing industry gradually to not-for-profit could leave this industry in private hands while simultaneously cutting huge and unnecessary costs in the health care system.

As the insurance industry gradually moves to a not-for-profit model, what incentive will they have to enter into tough negotiations with providers? With the exchanges as the marketplace, individuals will be constantly making price versus quality judgments and decisions.

Currently, a health provider's only incentive is to lobby for as high a reimbursement as possible, only moderated by their desire to be in as small a panel[2] as possible.

Insurers realize their tension point is having a panel of doctors and hospitals of sufficient size and quality, at a price point employers will purchase.

Employers need a panel employees find attractive. Insurers' leverage with providers is limited to the status, size, and reputation of the panel. Since employers must often satisfy an employee group with a wide variety of health needs and provider preferences, the insurers' leverage on price negotiations is muted.

The exchanges have the potential to change everything. We have noted, under an employer mandate, most corporations would move to pay a fine and dump their employees into the exchange. The speed of this conversion depends on the size of the fine. The lower this fee, the quicker the change.

Booz & Company, a global-management-and-strategy consulting firm, estimates 60 percent of the currently uninsured will enter the insurance market through an expanded Medicaid program. Another 28 percent will be covered, many with subsidies, by the new state exchanges. The remainder will get their coverage through employer groups now stimulated to provide coverage by the employer mandate.

Their analysis is that, while five to seven million employees will be moved by their employers to the exchange, the majority of employed Americans will continue to get their coverage through the traditional employer-sponsored plans.

I believe whether I am right or whether their prediction is more apt is entirely dependent on the level of the fine versus the cost of continuing to provide coverage. It will take only one employer in any industry to step out, drop coverage, and not suffer any consequences in employer morale or recruitment capabilities before the rest of the employers in that group will all follow suit. Once the dam breaks, the switch will occur rapidly.

There are two alternatives to an employer mandate. As a country, we can, of course, do nothing. This would condemn us to our current flight path. More and more employers are currently dropping health insurance simply because of cost, resulting in more uninsured. *The Bloomberg Report* notes the annual cost per employee, per year, is approximately $11,000.

The second alternative is considerable tax incentives. In my mind, the only viable alternative to encourage employer coverage is a combination of incentives and a mandate. The employers' net out-of-pocket expenses should be roughly the same whether they choose to pay the fine or provide health coverage to their employees.

Employers then would make the decision, not on economic grounds but on the importance of health insurance to their human resource platform, their recruiting practices, and their need for low turnover. Either way, employees have coverage and choice.

Physicians

The second major piece of our cost puzzle—what we pay for care—is subject to huge variation.

Industrial engineers know variation in any process always brings inefficiency and higher prices.

Standardization controls costs, as every successful manufacturer or retailer has learned. The variation in how we
treat patients with the same illness is huge and unexplainable. Experts have estimated 20 percent to 30 percent of
health cost is this unexplained variation.

Jack Wennberg of Dartmouth University, the major
researcher on medical variation, notes one-third of the
2.4 trillion dollars in annual health care expenditures is
wasted by unnecessary treatments, overpriced drugs, and
futile end-of-life care.

Intelligent use of evidenced-based medicine for many
chronic diseases represents a strategic opportunity. For
many prime diseases, experts have developed protocols to
move patients expeditiously through the health system.
Medical schools and specialty societies have determined
what pathways of care make the most sense.

Pathways help determine what medical decisions are
least influenced by doctor prejudices and which subject
the patient to the least risk, consistent with thoroughly
diagnosing and treating their problem. These protocols
should always allow the physician to go in another direction if the peculiarities of the patient dictate a change.

The patient should be financially motivated to understand their disease; they should be compliant with physician instruction, including changing behavior; and they
should follow the patient portion of the protocol.

If we ever hope to reduce variation and thus realize the
cost savings as a result, following the evidence is the only
solution. Fortunately, there are systems today that assist

the physician and the patient by giving them incentives to follow the protocols.[3]

There is a second variation in medical practice not related to physician preferences or prejudices.

This variation has simply to do with the lack of information between physicians, hospitals, and clinics. Records, in many cases, are still being kept in a handwritten format. Even where patient information has been automated, the systems do not talk to each other across and among provider groups.

For example, a patient on vacation shows up in a hospital emergency room in the middle of the night with chest pain. The ER doctor has no way of knowing the medication the patient has taken, no way of knowing what diagnostic tests have been performed, no way of knowing whether this patient had a recent coronary arteriogram, and no way of knowing the results.

In other words, except for the patient's memory, or perhaps locating the patient's cardiologist, the emergency room doctor is flying blind. As a result, tests get repeated, and perhaps expensive and redundant procedures are performed.

All of this is at great expense and risk to the patient. The data needed to avoid this unnecessary cost and risk is found elsewhere, in someone else's information system. It is simply not available at this moment of crisis.

An electronic record with a standard format, easily accessible to all who come into contact with a patient, would eliminate huge duplications and variation.

This data disconnect is universal and affects virtually every decision the physician must make. The *Journal of*

Health Affairs has estimated a shared electronic medical record could save approximately five percent of our total health bill.

Why does this seemingly easy fix elude us? I believe part of the problem is, again, incentives.

The software vendors have little incentive to standardize their products. Their systems are sold as a way for buyers to differentiate themselves from their competitors. Standardization would end this marketing ploy.

Hospitals should not compete on the sophistication of their information technology platform but on the quality of care.

This lack of standards means that for providers to be linked electronically, programming must be developed, which is often costly and not very effective.

This lack of data transparency makes it difficult for doctors to be effective. Data in a standard format, available real-time to every doctor irrespective of the treatment venue, should be the goal.

An airline pilot moving from American Airlines to Delta to fly a 747 has an easy transition as the technology is consistent and standard. Health care in America needs that same consistency for its physicians.

If we use the most conservative estimates of savings for improving overhead and taking unnecessary cost out of the system, we are beginning to see a significant difference.

Despite the power of evidenced-based medicine and enhanced electronic medical records, we also must change how physicians organize themselves. Standard fee-for-service practice is responsible for developing a physician culture of focusing on their patients. This culture has made being a physician in America one of the most rewarding professions. We treasure a personal relationship with our doctors.

But this mode of practice also has brought us variation that insures high-cost solutions to every problem. It has brought us a lack of collaboration that lets patient needs sometimes fall through the cracks simply because there is no forum that produces that very collaboration.

The *Patient Protection and Affordable Care Act* encourages experimentation with different models of physician organization. The Accountable Care Organization is envisioned to function very similarly to the Health Maintenance Organizations of an earlier decade.

Since there is a single payment to cover the health needs of a population for a defined period of time, the whole ball game changes. The physician incentive system is turned on its head. Since the payment is fixed for a period of time, gone is the incentive for physician income maximization, inherent in the fee-for-service system.

We have noted physicians are already beginning to reorganize themselves under corporate umbrellas, either as part of a hospital system or in large multi-specialty groups.

In a fixed-payment system, size is an advantage. Collaboration to keep costs down is essential for survival. Size means access to capital, which allows control of the diagnostic and treatment environment. Survival, in a fixed payment world, means physicians must have the capacity to collaborate on each patient's needs, tailored to their individual circumstances—providing what is needed, but only what is absolutely necessary.

The penalties for failure to collaborate and practice conservative medicine are severe. The pressures for physicians to move into groups to gain leverage, control of the entire spectrum of treatment options, and protect income are mounting.

Fewer new physicians are embracing private practice. Formation of Accountable Care Organizations only accelerates this natural movement. In addition, there are new requirements for the automation of their records, with which a physician's office must be compliant by 2015.

The cost of this conversion is often difficult for a small private practice to finance. Physicians with insufficient capital or the willpower to convert will be drawn into larger groups or hospital systems. Thus, the natural movement toward consolidation of medical practices coincides nicely with the switch of fee-for-service to fixed payment.

Under any scenario, more primary care doctors will be necessary. Even without health reform, the number of primary care physicians currently active will be insufficient to meet the needs of a rapidly maturing baby-boom population.

The number of primary care physicians has been kept artificially low due to their income levels, compared to their specialist colleagues.

It is my belief, in an Accountable Care Organization environment, the role of the primary care physician becomes critical. Their income, relative to the specialist, should begin to improve. Medical schools and residency programs should be encouraged to improve primary care output.

State Scope of Practice laws should be changed to allow alternative health professions, such as physician assistants or nurse practitioners, to extend their capabilities. To meet the needs of an aging population, we simply must allow more allied health providers at the point of patient contact. This expansion of responsibility would allow primary care physicians to spread their expertise across a wider boundary of patients.

One final physician incentive: across the country, thousands of caring physicians volunteer their time to see at-risk patients. These are most often the uninsured. We could substantially increase this volunteerism with one simple change.

If we gave physicians tax credits for their volunteer work, we would substantially increase the number of physicians willing to volunteer. With this relatively easy step, a sizable number of uninsured would gain access to medical care. If we add to these credits enhanced malpractice protection for volunteer work, we could draw thousands of retired physicians back to active practice in free clinics.

Between these two initiatives, a sizable number of uninsured would have, for the first time, access to care.

Interestingly, malpractice reform received only tepid acknowledgment in the *Patient Protection and Affordable Care Act*. If there is one singular element of our health care system that is unique, it must be our medical tort system. To control the cost side of the equation, this element must be addressed. In the grand scheme, relatively few doctors get sued. The cost of malpractice—often called professional liability coverage—is a small part of the overall cost picture of American health care.

However, the psychological impact of the threat of being sued is enormous. If every doctor believes he or she runs the risk of a lawsuit because of a test or procedure they chose not to do, the accelerator effect on cost is enormous. Doctors act on that belief, and because of that belief, numerous tests and procedures that might not otherwise have been done get ordered. The psychology of protecting oneself is a huge accelerator on the cost of care.

The typical response to this issue in various state legislatures is to pass limitations on damage rewards. Courts typically find this approach troubling and not infrequently declare such legislation unconstitutional. Any tort reform must first be fair to the injured patient.

There are two types of patient injuries caused by medical mistakes. First is the obvious serious mistake resulting in significant harm. An example is overdosing the patient with a lethal medication and resultant major harm to the patient.

The second type of mistake is less serious with little resultant harm to the patient. My premise is either way patients should ultimately have access to the court system, but this should be a system with some rationality that compensates patients for their identifiable harm.

First, I would propose an annuity system that allows the provider and the courts to calculate the present value of future payments to correct the harm that was done. This allows the offending provider to pay the true cost of future care year by year. The patient is protected by the establishment of an annuity.

I know this would work because the trial lawyers would hate it. They would prefer to multiply an inflated estimation of the cost of yearly care by the premise that the injured party lives to full lifetime expectancy. When you multiply this inflated standard by fifty to eighty years of life, we wind up with the huge jury awards, of which the trial lawyer gets 50 percent.

Second, all claims would first be reviewed by a panel of experts before it ever reached the courthouse. These medical experts would not have been associated in the past with plaintiffs or defendants. No one who has ever appeared as either a plaintiff or defense witness would be eligible to sit on these expert panels. The opinion of these panels would and could be introduced as evidence by either side during trial.

If the fault and the resultant harm are small, then a preset range of penalties could be awarded by a judge. If the fault is clear and the harm is significant, then a jury could decide. Either way, the judge or the jury would have the advantage of a disinterested group advising them as to harm and causality.

This system would replace much of the natural emotion and sympathies that juries now feel. These sympathies promote runaway verdicts even when the evidence suggests the health provider is not at fault. Patients still retain full access to the court system. The findings of this panel would certainly influence both sides to serious and speedy settlement discussions.

Hospitals

If allowed, hospitals could be a tremendous source for public health improvement. They have capital; geographic reach; a large, well-educated employee base; and organizational talent.

A review of the American Hospital Association's[4] website will reveal hospital organizations that have initiated some incredible services to improve community health.

The point is they currently have little incentive to do so. Yes, for the not-for-profits, justifying their tax exemption might be a motivating factor. However, that justification can be generally achieved by seeing charity patients in the emergency room.

I point with pride to my own organization's operation of a charter school for at-risk children. In fact, it can be argued that currently such efforts only detract from their real mission: beating their competitors.

If hospital executives were, in part, incentivized to cooperate with their competitors to improve public health, the resources brought to solve sometimes-intractable problems, such as teenage pregnancy, would be impressive. The combined strength of these organizations as collaborators, instead of just competitors, to serve the public good would be extraordinary.

It actually would not take much in the way of incentive to stimulate this collaboration. Tax incentives for for-profit hospitals or modest grants to not-for-profit hospital consortiums would stimulate a natural inclination of hospitals to pursue more of a community focus and less of a self-serving one.

The pressures of a more price-sensitive insurance exchange and a fixed-price reimbursement system would alter the hospital landscape. In this environment, there is significantly less incentive to duplicate high-cost technology and services that are often only marginally successful.

This new environment would force significant consolidation across the entire industry. There would be fewer, much larger hospital players whose primary incentive would be to rationalize their service offerings across their geography and eliminate those ineffective ones.

Changing insurance overhead would result in a 15 percent to 20 percent savings. Following the evidence and eliminating variation would produce another 20 percent to 30 percent savings. Having a transparent real-time information system and eliminating duplication of tests, medication, and procedures results in another five percent savings.

This retooling could save conservatively 40 to 50 percent of our costs. We could then make the argument there is already enough money in health care with these changes that we could accomplish our goal.

American Public

Perhaps the most difficult part of any reform plan is what to do with the uninsured who, for whatever reason, simply choose not to play.

Our national inclination as Americans is to simply say no one should be forced to buy a product they do not want. This is, of course, the basis of the numerous state lawsuits questioning the constitutionality of the individual mandate.

We know there are millions of Americans who simply consider themselves bullet proof, who do not trust insurance companies, or who are making a political statement by refusing to buy coverage. Their decision is, of course, facilitated by the fact that if they get sick or hurt, they can come to the emergency room and avail themselves of care, for which the rest of us will pay.

Our decision to ignore these people would be easy if we also could ignore their eventual health needs.

For instance, if we could leave our cyclist bleeding by the side of the road because he chose not to buy insurance he could afford, that would be the essence of free choice. The cyclist would then suffer the consequences of his decision.

What could be fairer? You choose not to buy insurance; that is your prerogative, but do not expect the rest of us to pick up the tab for your desire to exercise your individual rights.

But of course, our humanitarianism requires us to scrape him off the street, deliver him to a high-cost ER, and spend thousands of dollars to repair his broken body.

The Supreme Court will ultimately decide if we can be forced to buy a product we choose not to. The good sisters at Holy Trinity Catholic School in Dallas taught me God gave man the gift of free will. Because of that gift, the sisters said God eventually holds all of us accountable at judgment day for the choices we made. This is the consequence of the freedom of choice.

In most states, we can choose not to buy auto insurance, but we do not have the right to drive a car without it. If we choose to refuse to buy this insurance and drive a car anyway, we can be subject to a heavy fine.

Accordingly, what are the consequences of refusing health insurance?

While you might not find most physicians' offices open to you, nevertheless, the ER is never closed.

As long as the rest of us will pay for the exercise of your free will, then you, in effect, have a pass on the consequences of that decision.

There are, of course, two problems with this analogy. First, the auto insurance mandate is a state requirement. It does not have to pass the test of complying with our federal constitution. Second, the requirement for auto insurance is in essence to protect the other driver. There is no requirement for insurance to protect ourselves. The first casualty of this analogy may, in fact, point us to a conclusion that has real significance.

The individual mandate has merit for two basic reasons. First, it allows insurers to spread the risk of covering known losses, such as preexisting conditions. With the risk base spread over a larger pool, insurers have the capability of being inventive. They could offer a wide variety of plan options, such as preventive services, comforted by the knowledge that the premium base is spread more evenly. Second, it limits those who wish to game the system and play the rest of us as chumps. The principle argument against the mandate is instead a constitutional argument.

The conclusion then is to not make it a federal mandate. Perhaps we should rethink the whole reform effort as a solely federal effort. Would we have been better off with national legislation that set some worthy goals for the states to meet within a certain time frame on coverage for the uninsured? This type of federal legislation also could stipulate all the insurance reforms that are so popular in the *Patient Protection and Affordable Care Act.*

The states would then have to use the tools available to accomplish the reforms and the added additional coverage. It is in this context that a state mandate makes sense.

As in state auto insurance, the mandate would protect the rest of us from having our premiums impacted by those who would choose to be irresponsible. In this thought process, the states would be laboratories to accomplish reform. The federal government's role would be to set goals and requirements so the end points would be consistent across states.

For instance, a worthy goal would be coverage of 95 percent of the states' population by 2015. Penalties for failure to achieve the goal would be severe. How it would be done in detail would, could, and should vary by state. Each state's diversity and cultural preferences would come into play. The goal of comprehensiveness of coverage would be accomplished. Market pressures through the exchanges would act to constrain cost.

There is a story that famous heart surgeon Dr. Michael DeBakey was once challenged by an auto mechanic. He stated he and DeBakey did essentially the same work but that DeBakey made considerably more money. Reportedly, DeBakey's response was, "You're right, but I operate while the engine is still running." This is, in essence, our problem: to reform a health system while it is still running.

People still need care. Hospitals and physicians still need to perform their vital services. Insurers need to continue to perform their claims payment function. The system continues to function while all the time we look for substantial changes that clearly will upset some vested interest.

In this last chapter, I have presented fifteen ideas to strengthen our effort to realize the goal of covering more of our citizens while constraining costs, building on our strengths, recognizing our uniqueness, and challenging our preconceptions.

In summary, they are:

1. *Recommit to the Goal*: Stephen Covey, in his book *The Seven Habits of Highly Effective People,* emphasizes that smart people always begin with the "end in mind." A focus on where you want to end up is essential to any reform effort. I would suggest the original goal of coverage for all was a worthy objective. That objective should remain the primary connector for all of us as we debate, sometimes with great passion, the details of how we get to that goal.

2. *Public Debate*: I suggest we enter a period of at least a year's discussion of the toughest issues the American public faces. Unless we try to energize, inform, and listen to the American people about issues, such as the care of the elderly, then we are subject to the often-uninformed rantings of those among us with the largest megaphones.

3. *Stimulate the Emergence of a Not-For-Profit Insurance Industry*: It is time we recognize health insurance for

[margin handwriting: could it begin to...]

what it is not. It is not insurance. It is a payment mechanism. We should reward those who perform this claims processing function the quickest with fairness to both payer and provider. Under proper conditions, the marketplace will facilitate this conversion.

4. *Implement the Exchanges*: State-run exchanges have the ability to place some market dynamics into a field that has been traditionally very resistant to the laws of supply and demand. Properly designed and managed exchanges allow consumers to make price point versus quality decisions right at their kitchen table. This consumer power would ultimately control provider pricing.

5. *Give Employers Real Choice*: Based on their human resource needs, employers should have a difficult decision on whether to pay a fee and send their employees to an exchange or provide coverage themselves. It is my sense the fee should be slightly less than the cost of employer coverage. This then allows the employer the option of keeping their coverage if that relationship with their employees is vital to how they operate their business. Either way, employees get coverage.

6. *Implementation of Evidenced-Based Medicine*: To control the cost curve, we simply must control variation in the practice of medicine. Our incentive system should reward physicians for following the evidence.

Safeguards should allow physicians to opt out of protocols with a documented justifiable reason. We cannot allow significant unexplained differences in how patients with the same health issues and the same demographics continue to be treated markedly different from each other. We must take advantage of technology-driven incentive systems to insure we begin to control variation.

Similarly, patients should be financially incentivized to follow their own protocols of evidence-based medicine. There should be a reward system for both patients and physicians to be compliant with the nation's best thinking on how to deal with chronic disease.

7. *Standards for Information Technology*: Patient information on histories, physicals, medications, diagnostic tests, and hospital stays should be available real time to all legitimate providers with patient permission. Complicit in this recommendation is the requirement for a strong identity management system. The provider must know that the John Smith on his computer screen is, in fact, the John Smith sitting in front of him.

This suggests the maintenance of a population identifier similar to our Social Security number. We pay too high a price in redundant tests, duplicative medications, and repeat procedures to not begin to capture all our medical data either in a single repository or in local repositories that can communicate with each other. This will require standardization of information technology systems that vendors might find threatening. Nevertheless, the cost savings would be significant.

8. *Accelerate the Formation of Accountable Care Organizations*: While our fee-for-service system has served the medical profession very well, its time as the main payment mechanism may be at an end. It has allowed for a personal relationship with our physicians. However, we have to ask, are the perverse incentives we place on our physicians, that they do more rather than less, viable in a time of runaway health costs? There is a real question whether coverage for all and a fee-for-service system can coexist.

We need to put physicians into a collaborative environment so the reward system is based around keeping a patient healthy. Put simply, we need a compensation system that rewards doctors for doing only what is absolutely necessary for the patient's adequate care and nothing more.

Parenthetically, I believe that under ideal circumstances physicians need to continue to be at the top of the economic pyramid. Their training justifies it, and their importance to our lives and well-being mandates it.

9. *Physician Manpower*: With the wave of baby boomers reaching their senior years and with a whole class of people now possessing an insurance card, the physician manpower issue becomes critical.

We simply must increase the output of primary care physicians from our training programs. The Government Accounting Office estimates primary care physicians' residencies between 1995 and 2006 fell by more than one thousand, and currently only 45 percent of primary care residencies actually filled. At a time of our greatest need, we are clearly going in the wrong direction.

With the emergence of Accountable Care Organizations, the role of the primary physician will become more essential and thus their income relative to the specialists should become more equalized. Our medical schools should play a key role in elevating the status of a primary care physician. Key incentives could facilitate that transition. For example, loan forgiveness for young physicians choosing primary care could be accelerated over the loan requirements for those in specialty fields.

In addition, State Scope of Practice laws should be amended to allow allied health professionals, such as physician's assistants and nurse practitioners, even more freedom than they enjoy today. Historically, state medical associations have resisted the expansion of capabilities for allied health professionals. Their actions were driven by their desire to protect physician prerogatives. Such resistance is counterproductive in an age of severe shortages of physician talent, particularly among primary care physicians.

While working under the supervision of a physician, these allied health professionals could relieve the burden of this new influx of patients. Accordingly, organized medicine should abandon its sometimes knee-jerk reactions to such legislative changes.

10. *Clever Use of Tax Incentives*: We should reward our physicians for doing good things. Serving in the inner city, in a poor rural community, or volunteering in a free clinic are all acts of selfless humanitarianism. These noble efforts deserve recognition. I believe it would not take much in the way of incentive to inspire even more physicians to pursue this selfless path.

Simply saying we recognize, we honor, and we reward your efforts to help the underserved would be a game changer. The additional effect on a physician's natural motivation to help would be profound.

11. *Hospitals as Change Agents*: We need to get closer to the reason many of our hospitals were first conceived and started. Citizens of good will or religious organizations started many of our current hospitals for one simple reason: to serve humanity and their community.

Time, money, and natural competitiveness have led many to behave as if their current sole motivator is to be more financially successful than their competitor. While understanding that competition drives hospitals to improve their service, it also drives them to concentrate on the most highly compensated services and to eschew efforts at collaborating for the public good.

Some well-placed tax incentives and/or grants for community improvement would stimulate their natural and historic inclinations for public service. Doing so, we would avail our communities of the tremendous reservoirs of talent that reside within our hospitals.

12. *Serious Tort Reform*: Our effort to change physician incentives and to encourage the use of evidenced-based medicine will be held hostage unless there is serious tort reform. Standard efforts to simply limit the size of awards miss the point. If we are trying to change physician behavior and eliminate the fear that stimulates the over-ordering of tests and treatment, then we need to convince physicians their actions will first be judged by their peers. Expert panels accomplish this while allowing patients full access to the judicial system.

13. *States as Laboratories*: Opponents of the *Patient Protection and Affordable Care Act* describe it as the most ambitious federal power grab in history. Supporters were disappointed it did not go far enough by its failure to include a government option in the exchange. What it certainly failed to do was allow the states any significant ability to fashion an approach suited to their individual diversity.

Perhaps the place that could have used state collaboration was the area of the individual mandate. My position is the mandate makes imminent sense when it is combined with new requirements for covering preexisting conditions and unlimited lifetime reserves. To cover known risk requires that the healthy must be included with the ill to fairly spread that risk.

Also, from a simple fairness perspective, the lack of an individual mandate would allow many to take advantage of the system, and push the ultimate responsibility for the cost of the uninsured onto the rest of us who play by the rules. Unfortunately, making it a federal mandate brought in the whole constitutional question, which may prove to be its undoing.

How much better it would have been to set the coverage standard and let the states decide how to meet those requirements. My prediction is many states would have chosen the individual mandate as the prime opportunity to reach greater levels of insured coverage.

14. *Money Already in the System*: The old comedy bit, which do you want first, the good news or the bad news, applies here. The good news is there is already money in the system to cover the uninsured without significant new taxes. The bad news is it will be very hard to ply that money out of the health system without major commitments to change.

By converting our insurance industry to not-for-profit, insisting on the use of evidenced-based medicine, and investing in standards for information technology that digitizes all our medical records and requires standards to facilitate systems that easily communicate with each other, we can generate enough new money to do that which we set out to do in the first place. It will take a commitment to the goal and the mental toughness to stay the course.

15. *End of Life Care*: We simply have to get the dying thing right. Medicare now spends 25 percent of its budget on care delivered in the last year of the beneficiary's life. Of that amount, 40 percent is spent during the last thirty days. Clearly, significant dollars are devoted to futile care at the end of our lives.

While the decision concerning how our parents should spend their last few days on this earth is very personal, nevertheless, decisions are routinely being made that have nothing to do with dying with dignity.

Part of the issue may be that families are divorced from the economic consequences of the decisions they make regarding their beloved family members. Part of the issue may be the physician culture perceives death as the ultimate failure and stimulates recommendations for care that add little value to the quality of life and in no way postpone the inevitable.

Part of the answer may be that our inability to deal with our own deaths gets projected onto our parents. Traditionally, our tort system stimulates a full court medical press to every end-of-life experience when simple palliative pain relief may be the most humane decision.

Whatever the reason, a national debate on this issue is necessary. This debate must be held with love and compassion for those elderly whose time draws near without being a wedge issue in the next election cycle.

Our physicians should be encouraged—and compensated—for having these discussions with us and our loved ones.

Making this a partisan debate fixed on political grandstanding strikes me as the height of leadership irresponsibility.

You may find it curious I have said relatively little about wellness. The need for us to be good stewards of our own bodies is self-evident. Healthy employees are less expensive employees. Healthy elderly require less expenditure from the Medicare program. Society would be better off if its citizens ate less, smoked less, drank less, and exercised more.

The problem is, you cannot prove being a good steward of your body actually saves money. It is virtually impossible for an employer to calculate a return on investment on a fitness program for their employees. The benefits are so far in the future that any payback is difficult to realize. The reason Medicare and Social Security are going bankrupt is that its beneficiaries are too healthy and live too long.

We are the victims of our own success in public health, in the treatment of illnesses, and in new technology. The cynic might say if we keep you alive today, you will die of something more expensive to treat tomorrow.

If we gauge our success by lengthening life expectancy, then we are amazingly successful. As we have eliminated childhood diseases and improved the environment, we have extended our lives.

Those of us who improve our risk factors by exercising or by taking statin drugs to control our cholesterol continue to postpone the days of our own deaths.

It is clear the eighty-year-old of today is similar to the sixty-year-old of past generations. Is there a pre-programmed date to which, under ideal circumstances, humans could live? Might that be 120? Could that extension happen by the next generation?

While living to that advanced age might be attractive to us as individuals, the social costs are significant. Our aging population is already causing us to rethink our historic social contract. Our entitlement programs are already breaking under the weight of science's ability to extend life.

When should we retire? Are the mid-sixties simply too soon? What are the consequences of working into our seventies on the economy's ability to create sufficient jobs to support this new group of healthy elderly and those just beginning to enter the workforce in their twenties?

We know there are big savings to current health costs by reducing risk factors and by controlling variation of medical practice. This present savings, however, will come at the expense of creating a more costly patient in the future. If today's eighty is yesterday's sixty, then is tomorrow's one hundred today's eighty? If so, we need some serious conversation concerning the economic consequences of an aging population.

Each of us has a role to play in being good ambassadors for our own health. Each of us has a role to play in insuring that the least among us has access to adequate health services. Each of us has an opportunity to think deeply about his or her own life and, yes, his or her own death.

We have the obligation to discuss with our loved ones the difference in having a life and simply being alive. We have an obligation to be better informed and thoughtful about the health issues of our time. Recall the intense controversy in 2005 around removing the feeding tube of Terri Schiavo. Even members of Congress felt the need to interject their wisdom into this highly personalized decision. Perhaps the real debate should have been whether the feeding tube should have been inserted in the first place.

The point will be to have the capacity to discuss uncomfortable subjects while respecting a variety of opinions. Our doctors have an obligation to live up to the motivation that brought them to the study of medicine in the first place. Their desire is to make a real difference in patients' lives.

This motivation for some has been corrupted by self-serving opportunities for income advancement. Hospitals have an obligation to see that their ultimate mission is to be a force for community benefit.

Their motivation for survival does require a sense of competitiveness. That sense of competition should not substitute for the values that brought Catholic nuns across the plains in covered wagons to establish places of refuge for the sick and poor.

Our insurers have an obligation to understand they are not essential to the care process. Their function is to move money from those receiving care to those providing care. This function provides the grease necessary to keep the parts of the system in working order.

Though not essential for the care process, it is important the insurer's job be done with dispatch and fairness. While they need to be paid fairly for this claims adjudication function, it should not absorb 20 percent of every health care dollar.

Our policy makers have an obligation to help shape a system that provides care for more people while not bankrupting this country. This obligation has nothing to do with scoring political points. It has to do with serving the needs of their constituents. While it is easy to be very cynical over whether we can ever expect statesmanship from elected officials, I remain optimistic some will emerge.

If I am right, we have the resources currently to cover all our citizens reasonably and fairly. But we have neither the ability to solve today's issues nor tomorrow's impending crisis using the politics of the least common denominator.

We have always been a country as much concerned about the next generation as our own.

The question is, are we willing to continue that tradition?

Epilogue

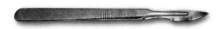

It's clear to me I have been especially critical of our politicians. This is perhaps a bit unfair. After all, they are the individuals who have stood the rigors of the election process and exposed themselves and their families to months of hard work and often harsh and undeserved criticism. They deserve our respect for having subjected themselves to perhaps the worst of all human endeavors: running for office. But it is the very rigors they face in the election cycle that make them often obtuse to acting on principle rather than political expediency

A smart lobbyist told me in reviewing any political initiative, politicians ask themselves three questions:

1. Will support of this initiative help get me reelected?

2. Will that support help me raise money from the interest groups supporting this initiative in order that I can finance my reelection?

3. What is the right thing to do?

Most politicians never get to the third question unless the initiative or legislation meets the test of the first two. This is unfortunate. It perhaps is the reason we have so few statesmen in elected office. With the physical effort and significant financial drain it takes to win an office, it is small wonder that once there, most people will do anything to remain there. It is exactly this self-serving compulsion that makes our Congress and the administration guilty of political malpractice.

Endnotes

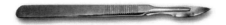

1. Routinely the carriers will pay out of network providers a significantly smaller amount, leaving the patient with a much greater private portion for the insured to finance. The patient then has a significant incentive to choose a hospital in the network, even if it means switching doctors.

2. A panel is the group of doctors and hospitals that have negotiated with the insurance companies for discounted fees in exchange for more patients to be directed to seek care from them.

3. For an education in one of the best of these, see *medencentive.com*.

4. American Hospital Association, see the section on McGaw and Nova Awards

Bibliography

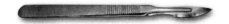

Abelson, Reed. "Insurers Push Plans That Limit Health Choices." *The New York Times* [New York] 18 July 2010, early ed.: 1. Print.

Ahlquist, Gary D., Paolo F. Borromeo, and Sanjay B. Saxena MD. "The Future of Health Insurance, Demise of Employer-Sponsored Coverage Greatly Exaggerated." *Booz Allen Hamilton: A Strategy and Technology Consulting Firm.* 18 Apr. 2011. Print.

American Hospital Association. "AHA Environmental Scan 2011." *American Hospital Association.* 2011. Print.

Bethea, MD, Charles F. *Age-Adjusted Death Rates for Total Cardiovascular Disease, Diseases of the Heart, Coronary Heart Disease, and Stroke by Year–United States 1900-1996. INTEGRIS Heart Hospital.* INTEGRIS Health. Web. 12 Nov. 2010. Print.

Bethea, MD, Charles F. *International CHD Mortality Trends in Men: 1968-2003. INTEGRIS Heart Hospital.* INTEGRIS Health. Web. 12 Nov. 2010. Print.

"Citizens' Health Care Working Group: Interim Recommendations." *UNT Libraries: CyberCemetery Home.* Citizens' Health Care Working Group. Print. 1 June 2006.

"Citizens' Health Care Working Group: Recommendations." *An American Dialogue.* Citizens' Health Care Working Group. Print. 2 March 2011.

Covey, Stephen R. *The 7 Habits of Highly Effective People: Restoring the Character Ethic.* New York: Free, 2004. Print.

"Dartmouth Atlas of Health Care." *Dartmouth Atlas of Health Care.* John Wennberg and Elliott Fisher. Web. 18 Apr. 2011. <http://www.dartmouthatlas.org/tools/downloads.aspx>.

Daschle, Thomas, Scott S. Greenberger, and Jeanne M. Lambrew. *Critical: What We Can Do about the Healthcare Crisis.* New York: Thomas Dunne, 2008. Print.

Dowd, Bryan, Steven Pizer, and Roger Feldman. "What Voters Look for in Health Insurance." *Ppionline.org.* Progressive Policy Institute, 18 May 2009. Web. 22 Dec. 2010. <http://www.ppionline.org>.

Emanuel, Ezekiel J., and Victor Robert Fuchs. *Healthcare, Guaranteed: A Simple, Secure Solution for America.* New York: PublicAffairs, 2008. Print.

Free Clinic Solutions and Georgia Free Clinic Network. *A Guide to National Health Care Reform for America's*

Free & Charitable Clinics. 1st ed. Atlanta, GA: Georgia Free Clinic Network, 2010. Print.

Friedman, Emily. "But They Said This Key Would Work: Coverage, Access and the Meaning of Insurance, Part 1." *Hhnmag.com.* HHN Magazine. Web. 11 Oct. 2010. <http://www.hhnmag.com>.

"From Courtship to Marriage, Part I: Why Health Reform is Driving Physicians and Hospitals Closer Together." *Magazine Article.* Pricewaterhouse Coopers LLP, Health Research Institute. Print. 2010.

Godges, John. "Third Opinion–A Leading Health Researcher Looks Beyond the Reform Debate." *Rand Corporation.* Rand Corporation, 2009. Web. 12 Nov. 2010. <http://www.rand.org>.

Greene, Jeff. "A Payment Reform and Provider Performance Rating System." *MedEncentive–Rewarding Better Health.* Print. 2011.

Hitt, Emma Ph.D. "Physician and Patients' Perceptions of Care, Knowledge Differ." 9 Aug. 2010. Print.

"How to Redesign Health Care." Rev. of *Magazine Article*, by Jay Parkinson. *Bloomberg Businessweek* 1 Feb. 2010. Print.

Jaspen, Bruce. "Malpractice Costs Top $55 Billion a Year in U.S., Harvard Study Says." *Chicago Tribune* [Chicago, IL] 8 Sept. 2010. Print.

Kendall, David B. "Fixing America's Health Care System." *PPi Policy Report* (2005). Print.

Kendall, David. "Health Care Costs and Malpractice Reform." *Ppionline.org*. Progressive Policy Institute, 1 Jan. 2008. Web. 22 Dec. 2010.

Levitt, Steven D., and Stephen J. Dubner. *Super Freakonomics: Global Cooling, Patriotic Prostitutes, and Why Suicide Bombers Should Buy Life Insurance*. 1st ed. New York, N. Y.: Harperluxe, 2009. Print.

Mechanic, Robert E., and Stuart H. Altman. "Payment Is A Good Place To Start." *Health Affairs*. Health Affairs. Web. 11 Nov. 2010. <http://content.healthaffairs.org>.

Mitchell, Jean M. "Utilization Changes Following Market Entry by Physician-Owned Specialty Hospitals." *Medical Care Research and Review*. Volume 64 Number 4. August 2007. Sage Publications. Print.

Morrison, Ian. "Flip the Switch." *Hhnmag.com*. HHN Magazine. Web. 9 July 2010. <http://www.hhnmag.com>.

Morrison, Ian. "In Search of the Next Economy." *Hhnmag.com*. HHN Magazine. Web. 2 Nov. 2010. <http://www.hhnmag.com>.

Newman, David H. *Hippocrates' Shadow*. New York: Scribner, 2009. Print.

Orlikoff, James E., and Mary K. Totten. "Health Care Reform: What's on the Horizon for Hospitals?" *Trustee Workbook* (2010). Print.

Osborne, David. "Outdated Ideology Could Derail Health Reform." *Progressive Policy Institute*. Web. 22 Dec. 2010.

Phend, Crystal. "National Health System No Cure for Mortality Disparities." *MedPageToday.com*. MedPage Today. Web. 12 Nov. 2010. <http://www.medpageto-day.com>.

Reid, T. R. *The Healing of America: a Global Quest for Better, Cheaper, and Fairer Health Care*. New York: Penguin, 2009. Print.

"Researchers Peg Malpractice Costs at Over $55 Billion." Rev. of *Magazine Article*, by Jennifer Lubell. *Modernhealthcare* 7 Sept. 2010. Print.

Responsible Reform for the Middle Class. "The Patient Protection and Affordable Care Act." 5 Jan. 2010. Print.

"Reinventing Healthcare for the 21st Century." *Magazine Article, by* Rita, Paul da and Tvede-Jensen, Lars. Pricewaterhouse Coopers *Gridlines 2010*. Print.

Schile, Rob. "The Six Major Themes of Health Care Reform." *Larsonallen.com*. LarsonAllen LLP. Web. 11 Nov. 2010.

"Top Health Industry Issues of 2011, Health Reform Prompts Industry Players to Undergo Makeovers." *Magazine Article.* Pricewaterhouse Coopers LLP. Print. 2010.

"Why Most Employers Will (and Should) Retain Their Health Care Plan after 2013." Rev. of *Magazine Article*, by Brad Warrick. *National Healthcare Reform Magazine* 19 Oct. 2010. *Http://www.healthcarereformmagazine.com.* National Healthcare Reform Magazine. Web. 11 Nov. 2010.

Wolf, Richard. "Doctors Limit New Medicare Patients– USATODAY.com." *News, Travel, Weather, Entertainment, Sports, Technology, U.S. & World– USATODAY.com.* Web. 18 Apr. 2011. <http://www.usatoday.com/news/washington/2010-06-20-medicare_N.htm>.

Young, Alison. "Case Against Blue Cross Shows Difficulty of Cutting Health Costs." *USA Today* [Pontiac, MI] 10 Nov. 2010. Print.